Insulin Pumps and Continuous Glucose Monitoring 2ND EDITION

A USER'S GUIDE TO EFFECTIVE DIABETES MANAGEMENT

FRANCINE R. KAUFMAN, MD, WITH EMILY WESTFALL

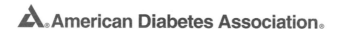

Director, Book Publishing, Abe Ogden; *Managing Editor,* Rebekah Renshaw; *Acquisitions Editor,* Victor Van Beuren; *Project Manager,* Wendy Martin; *Production Manager and Composition,* Melissa Sprott; *Cover Design,* Vis-à-Vis Creative Concepts; *Printer,* Data Reproductions

Printed in the United States of America
1 3 5 7 9 10 8 6 4 2

The suggestions and information contained in this publication are generally consistent with the *Standards of Medical Care in Diabetes* and other policies of the American Diabetes Association, but they do not represent the policy or position of the Association or any of its boards or committees. Reasonable steps have been taken to ensure the accuracy of the information presented. However, the American Diabetes Association cannot ensure the safety or efficacy of any product or service described in this publication. Individuals are advised to consult a physician or other appropriate health care professional before undertaking any diet or exercise program or taking any medication referred to in this publication. Professionals must use and apply their own professional judgment, experience, and training and should not rely solely on the information contained in this publication before prescribing any diet, exercise, or medication. The American Diabetes Association—its officers, directors, employees, volunteers, and members—assumes no responsibility or liability for personal or other injury, loss, or damage that may result from the suggestions or information in this publication.

⊗ The paper in this publication meets the requirements of the ANSI Standard Z39.48-1992 (permanence of paper).

ADA titles may be purchased for business or promotional use or for special sales. To purchase more than 50 copies of this book at a discount, or for custom editions of this book with your logo, contact the American Diabetes Association at the address below or at booksales@diabetes.org.

American Diabetes Association
2451 Crystal Drive, Suite 900
Arlington, VA 22202

DOI: 10.2337/9781580406604

Library of Congress Cataloging-in-Publication Data
Names: Kaufman, Francine Ratner, author. | Westfall, Emily, author. | American Diabetes Association.
Title: Insulin pumps and continuous glucose monitoring : a user's guide to effective diabetes management / Francine R. Kaufman and Emily Westfall.
Description: 2nd edition. | Arlington : American Diabetes Association, [2017] | Includes bibliographical references and index.
Identifiers: LCCN 2017016617 | ISBN 9781580406604 (paperback)
Subjects: LCSH: Insulin pumps. | Diabetes--Treatment. | Insulin--Therapeutic use. | Blood sugar monitoring. | Patient education. | BISAC: HEALTH & FITNESS / Diseases / Diabetes.
Classification: LCC RC661.I63 K38 2017 | DDC 616.4/622--dc23
LC record available at https://lccn.loc.gov/2017016617

CONTENTS

ACKNOWLEDGMENTS

We would like to acknowledge Professor Harry Keen for his contributions to insulin pump therapy. Professor Keen died at the age of 87 on April 5, 2013. He was a visionary in realizing what insulin pump therapy could do to improve the lives of individuals dependent on insulin treatment. We would also like to acknowledge Professor John Pickup for his innumerable studies and scientific manuscripts that helped advance the field of diabetes technology over the last four decades. In addition, the passing of Alfred E. Mann on February 25, 2016, was a loss of a great scientific and business leader. Alfred Mann founded the first successful diabetes technology company that made insulin pumps and continuous glucose monitors. Mann envisioned that these could be combined to automate insulin delivery to improve the lives of people with diabetes—something we are just realizing while writing this second edition. Mann was 90 years old at his death.

We have had many reviewers, including Kelly Joy, Gail Vanairsdale, Julie Schmaderer, Linda Burkett, and Theodora Padron. Their advice and editing were invaluable.

As always, we are inspired by our patients and their families, as well as our own families.

INTRODUCTION

This is the second edition of *Insulin Pumps and Continuous Glucose Monitoring: A User's Guide to Effective Diabetes Management.* It was imperative that we update this book because the field of diabetes technology has advanced so rapidly over the last 3 years. There have been so many enhancements to insulin pump therapy since the first insulin pump in the early 1980s. The first pump was jokingly referred to as the "big blue brick," and it weighed several pounds. The insulin-filled syringe was on the outside of the pump, the pump used a butterfly needle (the needle commonly used for intravenous delivery of medications) placed in the subcutaneous tissue, and, for the most part, it could only be used in the hospital setting. However, despite its many drawbacks, most felt the pump was a great advancement for patients, who benefitted from the continuous delivery of basal insulin and from the intermittent boluses that were given to match their food intake and to correct an abnormal blood glucose level when indicated. Over the ensuing 30 years, we have all witnessed incredible advances in the understanding of what happens to the cells of the body as the result of the diabetes process. We have seen tremendous breakthroughs in diabetes drug discovery, including the development of a myriad of insulin analogs, some now coupled with other injectable and oral medications, and rapid advances in glucose monitoring technology. We have determined better ways to deliver diabetes education and support, and we continue to combat discrimination against people with diabetes. And most importantly for this book, today we have insulin pumps that are small, fast, and smart, and we have continuous glucose monitors (CGMs). CGMs can give information retrospectively or in real time to help with diabetes management decisions. CGM data can be transmitted to secondary screens through the cloud so the patients can view their own data more discreetly or send it to a family member or care provider in real time for additional help. In some devices, the pump and the CGM work together in a single system.

These integrated systems have allowed for the CGM to stop insulin delivery at either a preset or at a predicted low glucose threshold. "Artificial pancreas" systems that automate insulin delivery have been evaluated in a series of clinical trials, and a hybrid version is now approved for commercial release for people with diabetes.

When you or your child were diagnosed with diabetes, you might have felt that you embarked on a new, different life journey. To succeed on that journey, you need to effectively manage your diabetes so that the maximal amount of time is spent with glucose levels in the target range, and the minimum amount of time is spent in the low or high range. To accomplish this, you, with the help of your family and friends, must track glucose levels to be able to deliver insulin in a manner that closely resembles how your body produced and used insulin before you were diagnosed. Often, the best way to achieve this is to use an insulin pump. This step is now increasingly accompanied by using a CGM, either as a stand-alone device or integrated with the insulin pump. Integrated systems now allow for automation of insulin delivery and serve as the platform for the artificial pancreas. These technologies—although not really that much more complicated than your smartphone, computer with continually updated systems, or computerized, connected home devices—do require basic understanding, training, and follow-up adjustment to help improve diabetes outcomes.

The purpose of this book is to give you practical tips, including the knowledge and the skills to optimize insulin pump therapy and continuous glucose monitoring, if that is what you and your health care provider decide is best for you or your child. This book will walk you through everything from choosing the right pump or CGM for you, to how to download and review your settings and how to use your pump and/or CGM for effective diabetes care through daily activities, travel, school, or college. The future of pumps and CGM technology in diabetes care is also addressed. If you already have an insulin pump and feel confident with basal rates and bolus settings, you might want to review Section 2, The Nitty-Gritty about Pumps, and focus your attention on sections 3 and 4. If you are looking for information about CGMs, focus your attention on Section 3, Uploads, GGM, and Closing the Loop. The goal is to enable you to make your journey through life with diabetes as successful and as free from short- and long-term complications, and with as minimal burden, as possible.

SECTION 1: THE BASICS

The goal of Section 1 is to review the basic physiology of glucose control and what occurs when someone has diabetes. To understand what you are striving for, you must also be aware of glucose and A1C targets. The central principles of how diabetes is now managed are supported by a series of important research studies. The critical ones, such as the Diabetes Control and Complications Trial (DCCT) and important research studies concerning insulin pumps, CGMs, and integrated sensor-augmented pumps, with or without automated features, are reviewed so that you understand the evidence surrounding the recommendations for meticulous diabetes control.

The insulin pump is a small mechanical device worn by someone who has diabetes and who is treated with insulin. The insulin pump helps facilitate diabetes control and lifestyle flexibility. Insulin enters the body from the pump either after flowing down the tubing into a small cannula (a soft tube) or a small needle placed under the skin, or through "tubeless" pumps placed straight onto the body with a small needle automatically inserted. Most people with type 1 diabetes and many with type 2 diabetes who require intensive insulin therapy use basal-bolus regimens, and the benefits of basal-bolus therapy will be outlined. In addition, you will see how you can balance insulin administration, food, and activity with greater ease while using an insulin pump. The importance of glucose monitoring with blood glucose meters or CGM systems will be stressed. The importance of having glucose data, seeing patterns and trends, and using alerts and alarms will be explained as a way to facilitate diabetes management.

SECTION 2: THE NITTY-GRITTY ABOUT PUMPS

Section 2 gets into the practical aspects of insulin pump therapy. The components and features of the pump are described, emphasizing the pump's bolus calculator and many other advanced features, perhaps the most important of which is calculating something called insulin on board (IOB), or active insulin. Sections on both basal and bolus insulin delivery cover all aspects, from determining your initial pump settings to how to adjust settings over time. As you read through this section, it should become obvious that adjustment of the regimen is required throughout your diabetes journey, since factors such as growth, weight, activity, stress, and lifestyle habits change over time. Because food is a critical element in diabetes management, there is a detailed discussion of carbohydrates, protein, and fat; understanding how to read food labels; and ways to assess your portions. One of the true challenges in diabetes management is adjusting insulin and carbohydrate intake for planned and unplanned physical activity. To succeed with insulin pump therapy, it is critical to understand infusion sets, how they differ, and what you need to consider in making the decision about which set you want to use. An in-depth review of principles to manage exercise is given in this section.

SECTION 3: UPLOADS, CGM, AND CLOSING THE LOOP

Section 3 will help you understand how important it is to upload data from pumps and CGMs. These uploads can be used to help you understand your patterns and trends and also to make adjustments in your therapies. The basics of CGM will be described, including its components, how the interstitial glucose compares to the blood glucose, and how to use CGM to improve your diabetes outcomes. Having glucose values displayed continuously and the ability to see trends in glucose levels can help you avoid serious highs and lows. The latest advance in commercially available technology, the hybrid closed-loop system, will be discussed so that you understand how CGM data drive some aspects of insulin delivery.

SECTION 4: ILLNESS, TRAVEL, AND SCHOOL

Section 4 describes how special circumstances can influence your diabetes care. Although diabetes management can be challenging when you are at home, feeling well, and following your standard routine, special circumstances can make diabetes management more challenging. Situations like illness, traveling (particularly across time zones), or going off to school or college can affect glucose control. Understanding how to adjust your regimen and what to do with your glucose numbers is reviewed in this section. This information will include concepts of advanced pump therapy.

SECTION 5: ADJUSTING TO INSULIN PUMP AND CGM THERAPIES

Section 5 covers the developmental capabilities of children with regard to managing pumps. Partnering with schools and child care facilities is critical. With cloud-based connectivity, parents are now capable of monitoring their children's glucose levels even when they are not together. You should have realistic expectations of what your child can do with his or her increasing self-management skills. If you don't know what is reasonable, then you might push or hold back your child too much in the quest for independence. Your child's independence is your ultimate goal. When you begin pump and/or CGM therapies, it is like learning about diabetes all over again. You will concern yourself with more insulin dosages and settings, and you will have the ability to continually assess your glucose levels throughout the day and night. When you first start using devices, you may end up thinking about diabetes almost all of the time. This process can cause stress in and of itself. There are critical issues in accepting—and ultimately succeeding with—pump and CGM therapies. These include deciding whom to tell about your pump and CGM, getting used to being attached to one or two devices, and learning how your body image might be affected.

This section concludes by discussing the future and how diabetes technology will continue to advance and will describe the next steps in the automation of insulin delivery beyond automatic insulin shutoff devices and the hybrid closed-loop systems of today. The next step, a fully closed-loop or "artificial pancreas" system, should result in near-perfect control of glucose levels without much human intervention. The future is bright, and sharing its promise with you will conclude the book.

The goal of this book is to help you understand why you or your child might want to use an insulin pump and a CGM, to give you the skills to use them, and to help you optimize your or your child's journey with diabetes. Learning to master an insulin pump or CGM may seem overwhelming at the beginning, but these skills can become second nature in no time at all.

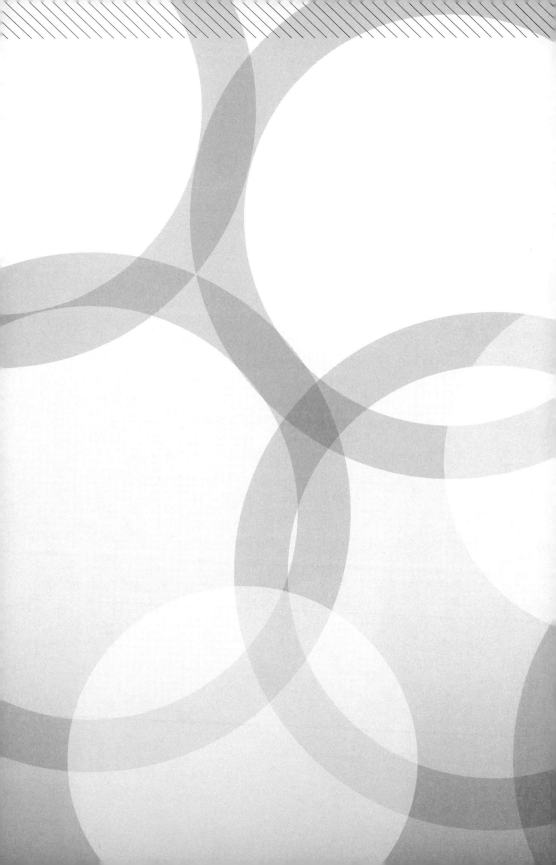

SECTION 1:
THE BASICS

IN THIS CHAPTER

CHAPTER 1

WHAT YOU NEED TO KNOW ABOUT DIABETES

REMEMBERING BACK TO DAY ONE

I bet you can remember the day you found out you or your child had diabetes. It is likely that you knew something was wrong for a few days—maybe even weeks—before the diagnosis was made, but you thought it was the flu or a new phase in your life or in your child's development. It is possible you even called your doctor and were told that the problem would go away soon and that there was likely nothing to worry about. Obviously, that wasn't the case.

Some children, teens, and adults are diagnosed with diabetes very early in the process, before they become sick. Some are screened for the presence of the antibodies or genes associated with type 1 diabetes because they have a family member with diabetes and they find out they are at risk of developing diabetes before they even have symptoms. Some are diagnosed only after they become seriously ill. But most have some, if not all, of the typical signs and symptoms of type 1 diabetes: frequent urination, increased thirst, weight loss, and fatigue. These signs and symptoms occur because the pancreas can no longer make enough insulin. Without enough insulin, multiple problems occur with metabolism within the body.

And now remember how remarkable it was just a few days after you were given insulin by injection or through an intravenous infusion (an IV). You were back to your usual self—active, hungry, gaining weight, and learning all about diabetes.

Look back at the first tasks you were asked to do: you had to start to give insulin shots and check blood glucose levels before you had

I give this Daily Schedule Sheet to my new patients.

DAILY TASKS

Test blood glucose
Determine insulin dose: # grams carb _____ + correction _____
Give insulin
Eat breakfast

Test blood glucose* (This should be 2–2½ hours after last meal)

*If your child would like to eat a snack at this time, you would:
    Determine insulin dose: # grams carb _____ + correction ____
    Give insulin
    Have child eat snack

Test blood glucose
Determine insulin dose: # grams carb _____ + correction _____
Give insulin
Eat lunch

Test blood glucose* (This should be 2–2½ hours after last meal)
*If your child would like to eat a snack at this time, you would:
    Determine insulin dose: # grams carb _____ + correction ____
    Give insulin
    Have child eat snack

even had a chance to adjust to the fact that you had diabetes. In those first days, you were mostly asked to read, study, and listen to lectures about this disease. You must have felt overwhelmed as it became apparent you were expected to become an expert, something that took us (and all our health-care-provider friends) years and years to accomplish.

Just like the example here, you were likely given a list of things to do and a schedule of when to do them. But essentially, by this time, you were aware that every day you needed to:

1. Take insulin to be able to metabolize food (mainly carbohydrate) and control the release of glucose from body stores

Before 4:30 P.M. call the diabetes team

Test blood glucose
Determine insulin dose: # grams carb _____ + correction _____
Give insulin
Eat dinner

Test blood glucose* (This should be 2–2½ hours after last meal)

*If your child would like to eat a snack at this time, you would:
    Determine insulin dose: # grams carb _____ + correction _____
    Give insulin
    Have child eat snack

At **12:00 A.M. (midnight)**, test blood glucose

At **3:00 A.M.**, test blood glucose

Give basal insulin at _____ daily

Manage exercise by measuring glucose before and after activity; take extra glucose as needed.

2. Measure glucose levels throughout the day and night to determine whether insulin doses are working properly

3. Eat a healthy and balanced diet, understand the quantity and quality of food, and couple food with taking insulin

4. Be physically active and understand the role of activity in glucose management.

Do see how far you have come from those first days? You have come far enough to now use or consider using an insulin pump and a continuous glucose monitor (CGM)—and to stay committed to doing what you can to optimize your journey with diabetes.

UNDERSTANDING THE BASICS ABOUT INSULIN

In a person who does not have diabetes, the body is designed to control glucose levels in the blood in a very narrow range. Although there are fluctuations of glucose levels throughout the day and night, generally glucose levels fall between 70 and 140 mg/dL— highest after eating and lowest after fasting (not eating). Insulin is secreted to keep the glucose that is released from your food moving into your body's cells. In the cells, glucose is used as fuel. Insulin also promotes storage of nutrients as a future energy source and helps prevent the liver from releasing glucose at inappropriate times, such as when you have just eaten.

Insulin is naturally secreted in two ways: 1) **background (called basal insulin)**, and 2) **surges (called bolus insulin)**.

1. **Background (or basal) insulin** controls the glucose levels between meals and overnight. It is mainly acting to help regulate how much glucose is released from the stores in the liver (where it is stored as glycogen). The release of glucose from the liver between meals is critical for providing energy so the body's cells can

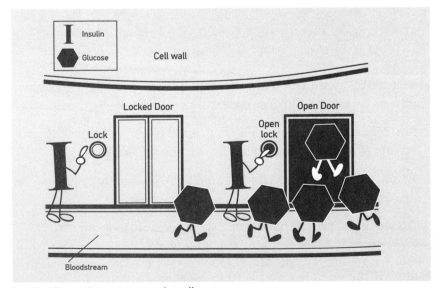

Insulin allows glucose to enter the cells.

function. Without enough background or basal insulin, your liver would release too much glucose into the bloodstream and your cells would not be able to use it for energy. This scenario could result in very high blood glucose levels. Additionally, without background insulin, the liver will start to produce acidic ketone bodies from the breakdown of fat. Your body is able to use fat as energy when there is not enough insulin around. Like sugar, these ketone bodies can be measured in the blood and in the urine. As ketones build up in the bloodstream, there is the risk of developing diabetic ketoacidosis (known as DKA). DKA is potentially a very dangerous condition.

2. **Surge (or bolus) insulin** occurs at mealtime. As glucose levels rise from meals, the pancreas responds with a large increase in insulin release, so the glucose can be stored for use by the body's cells. In the human body without diabetes, these surges are very precise: eat more, and more insulin is released; eat less, and not as much is released.

With diabetes (always in type 1 and sometimes in type 2), the ability to release enough insulin is lost. Since the discovery of insulin, replacement insulin therapy has evolved into the modern system we have today. The older system used a fixed approach to insulin replacement (although this is sometimes still used today).

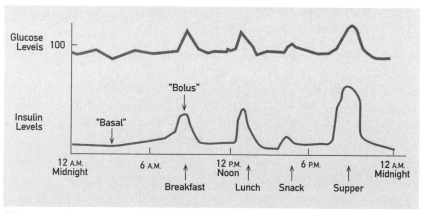

24-hour insulin and glucose profile in a person without diabetes, with the peak glucose <140 mg/dL.

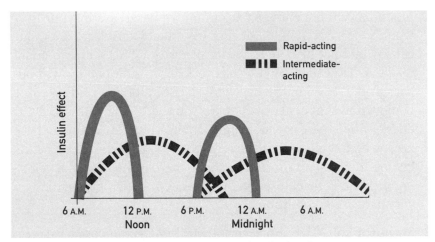

Two shots: a combination of intermediate- and rapid-acting insulins.

This figure shows one way to implement the fixed approach. The person with diabetes takes two shots a day. Each shot is a combination of intermediate- and rapid-acting insulin. As you can see, this approach is not very flexible. For example, if you eat dinner before 6:00 p.m., you won't have a bolus to cover the blood glucose rise. You could take your mixed shot earlier to cover the meal, but then you might not have any insulin in your system overnight. If you eat early but take your shot at the regular time, then you could have a high that is untreated.

Although you took only one to three shots a day, you had to take injections at set times and in set amounts. You had to eat the same amount of food at the same time every day, and you had to exercise at the same time every day. With this old way, keeping glucose in the target range was difficult for people with type 1 diabetes. And there was no flexibility in life. Essentially, your life had to fit into the diabetes regimen. The diabetes regimen controlled you.

The newer way to treat diabetes is with flexible regimens: multiple daily injections (MDI) or insulin pump therapy. These newer, flexible systems more closely mimic the way the pancreas normally produces and releases insulin. Flexible insulin regimens mimic background insulin and surges of insulin. They allow you to deliver insulin in doses to match your food intake and give you flexibility in how much you eat and when you eat it. You can be active when you want, and with an insulin pump, you can decrease basal insulin to avoid hypoglycemia. You can sleep when you want, wake up late, and travel around the globe with the flexibility to change from one

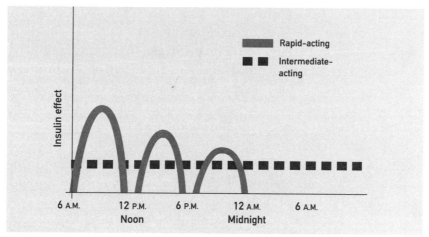

How an MDI regimen covers insulin requirements over the course of a day.

This figure shows how MDI covers insulin requirements over a 24-hour period. Because your basal and bolus insulins aren't tied together, you can take the bolus shot when you need it, giving you more flexibility in your lifestyle.

day to the next. When this is coupled with a glucose sensor measuring glucose levels every 5 minutes and a CGM, and if there is automated insulin delivery as is seen in some of the newer systems, flexible insulin regimens are effective in glucose management.

UNDERSTANDING THE TRANSITION FROM INJECTIONS TO PUMPS

When you were first diagnosed with diabetes, you were likely taking multiple injections of insulin every day, measuring blood glucose before meals and at bedtime (at a minimum), or wearing a continuous glucose sensor. Although it is possible that you were taking two or three injections (perhaps using NPH insulin), it is much more likely you started on MDI if you were diagnosed in the last number of years. With MDI, you use rapid-acting insulin and long-acting or basal insulin. These two different kinds of insulins have different jobs, but both work to keep your glucose in the target range.

Basal insulin is given as one or two shots each day, and it activates slowly after injection. This means that some amount of insulin will always be present in the blood. The blood can then bring insulin to the cells throughout the body, and glucose can then enter the cells, where it is converted into energy. In the liver, insulin helps regulate the slow release of stored glucose to meet the energy needs of the body's cells between meals and during the night.

Bolus insulin is given as rapid-acting insulin. It is activated much faster after injection and brings the large amount of glucose from your meals into your body's cells. There, glucose can be used right away for energy or stored for later use. Boluses with rapid-acting insulin can also be used to decrease a high blood glucose level. These doses are called "correction boluses."

The difference between an insulin pump and MDI is that an insulin pump just uses rapid-acting insulin to do both jobs of basal and bolus. The basal rates on the pump replace the basal or long-acting insulin injection in MDI. The pump basal rates allow for a small, almost continuous release of insulin. Boluses are given at meals and for correction. And these replace the mealtime and correction shots in the MDI regimen.

KNOW YOUR GLUCOSE AND A1C TARGETS

What is the ultimate goal of diabetes treatment? The goal is to effectively manage diabetes day to day, so that glucose levels are in the right range—known as the target range—as much as possible to avoid highs and lows. Keeping glucose levels in the target range minimizes your risk of short- and long-term complications. The target range for glucose is different at different times of the day. For example, in the morning when you haven't eaten for several hours (fasting), your target will be lower than it is after meals, when blood glucose is highest. Overnight, when you are sleeping, your target may be higher than the fasting range to protect you from hypoglycemia.

The normal fasting blood glucose for an individual (who is not pregnant) without diabetes is 70–100 mg/dL. For people with diabetes, the American Diabetes Association generally recommends a

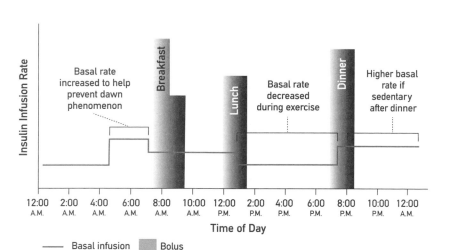

When you use an insulin pump, your basal rate and boluses are customized to more closely mimic how the body releases its own insulin. Both the basal infusion and the boluses are made with rapid-acting insulin.

fasting plasma glucose level of 80–130 mg/dL and after meals less than 180 mg/dL. In general, younger children have slightly higher targets for their glucose levels. In addition, there are a number of conditions that might lead the diabetes team to suggest higher targets, such as having repeated low blood glucose (hypoglycemia), being unaware of the symptoms of hypoglycemia (referred to as hypoglycemia unawareness), or having advanced diabetes complications or other diseases. You should discuss this with your diabetes team and find out what your target range glucose levels should be throughout the day, understanding that your target range should be individualized for you, and that it likely will change over time, as you age and as other conditions develop. Pregnancy, illness, and other acute conditions can change your target range; these topics will be discussed in detail later in the book.

Similarly, you should be aware of the target range for your HbA$_{1c}$ test (often called "A1C" for short). A1C measures the percentage (%) of your hemoglobin molecules (a protein in red blood cells) that have glucose attached to them. The higher your average glucose levels day after day, the higher your A1C. It gives you a good picture of what your glucose levels have been in general over the past several months. A1C should be measured every 3–6 months, and you should know what your level is each time it is taken. A1C is often referred to as the diabetes report card. By seeing if your A1C is in the target range set by your diabetes team, you can tell if your diabetes control is optimal.

In addition to specific glucose levels and A1C, there are many other important diabetes outcomes. Time spent in the target range, particularly when a glucose sensor is worn, or the amount of time in the hypoglycemic or hyperglycemic range, as well as measures of diabetes burden, are important for you to consider as your journey with diabetes continues.

RESEARCH SUPPORTING MDI, INSULIN PUMP THERAPY, AND CGM

There have been a lot of research studies in the fields of MDI and insulin pump therapy, as well as CGM and automated insulin delivery features. Most studies suggest that advancing diabetes technology has potential benefits in diabetes care. Here are some studies that have helped us better understand how to manage diabetes and how MDI and particularly insulin pump therapy can be a useful tool.

Diabetes Control and Complications Trial (DCCT)

Before the mid-1990s, someone with type 1 diabetes would take one (maybe two or, rarely, three) insulin injections per day. Back then, regular, NPH, lente, and ultralente insulins were in use. Except for NPH and regular, these other insulin preparations are not avail-

Age	Before meals	Bedtime/overnight	Postprandial
Children and adolescents	90–130 mg/dL	90–150 mg/dL	
	(5.0–7.2 mmol/L)	(5.0–8.3 mmol/L)	
Adults (nonpregnant)	80–130 mg/dL		<180 mg/dL
	(4.4–7.2 mmol/L)		(10.0 mmol/L)

Blood Glucose Targets for Children, Teens, and Adults
Taken from the *American Diabetes Association Standards of Medical Care in Diabetes—2017.*

able today. Insulin doses weren't adjusted from one day to the next, which meant that people had to follow a strict eating plan and physical activity regimen. That meant you couldn't skip breakfast, you couldn't delay having lunch, and if you routinely had a snack in the afternoon, you had to eat one even if you weren't hungry! Although you might have taken fewer shots, the trade-off in having a fixed diet and activity pattern wasn't worth it—and more importantly, this regimen led to inadequate diabetes control.

The Diabetes Control and Complications Trial (known as the DCCT) was a 9-year study. When the results were reported in 1993, the concept of how diabetes should be managed was changed forever. The investigators proved that tighter glucose control using MDI (three or more shots per day) or insulin pump therapy was better than conventional therapy at lowering A1C and reducing the risks of developing diabetes complications.

The DCCT conclusively showed that blood glucose control matters. Although the youngest participants in the DCCT were 13 years old when they entered the study, the overall results of the DCCT have been generalized to all of type 1 diabetes: optimal blood glucose control is the most effective way to reduce the long-term microvascular complications of diabetes.

Over 1,400 people with type 1 diabetes took part in the study. They were divided among two groups: one for intensive management and the other for conventional therapy (the way diabetes used to be managed). The intensive group used MDI (three or more shots per day) or an insulin pump. This group also received a great deal of support from the study teams. At the end of the DCCT, the people who used MDI had an average A1C level of 7.2%. Individuals receiving conventional therapy took one or two shots a day and did not have blood glucose targets or extra support from the study teams. Their average A1C level was 9.1%. Nine years later, people in the intensive group had fewer early signs of eye, kidney, and nerve problems than people in the conventional group. This result was a stunning discovery. However, the other lesson from the DCCT was that lowering A1C levels increases the risk of low blood glucose (hypoglycemia).

Epidemiology of Diabetes Interventions and Complications (EDIC) study

After the DCCT concluded in 1993, a follow-up study began, and it is still running today. The study is called Epidemiology of Diabetes Interventions and Complications (EDIC), and almost all of the DCCT participants entered into it. In the EDIC study, all of the participants went back to their usual health care team visits, and they were no longer cared for under a strict research protocol. Because of the powerful results of the DCCT, the EDIC participants and their health care teams tried to improve everyone's A1C. Individuals who had previously been in the intensive group had their A1C value increase, mainly because they no longer had all the support they received during the DCCT. People in the conventional group had their A1C value decrease because they saw the positive effects of intensive diabetes management. As a result, both groups achieved A1C levels around the 8% range. In the first 9 years of the EDIC study, participants previously assigned to the intensive group had a significant (57%) reduction in the risk of heart attack, stroke, or cardiovascular death compared with individuals previously in the conventional group. By 2009, participants who had been in the intensive group had lower rates of eye disease, kidney disease, and cardiovascular disease when compared with those in the conventional group. This result implied that there were benefits of having had intensive management and improved A1C levels, even if it was years before. In 2016, another report was published from the EDIC study concerning electrocardiogram (ECG) heart tracings. This report showed that a history of a higher A1C was a risk factor for having abnormalities on the ECG. This finding again underscored

LESSONS FROM THE DCCT AND EDIC STUDY

After 30 years of diabetes, fewer than 1% of participants in the intensive group had become blind, required kidney replacement, or had an amputation because of diabetes.

the benefits of intensive glycemic control in people with type 1 diabetes, which was shown to persist for decades.

Other Studies and Guidelines

Many studies have evaluated insulin pump therapy compared to MDI. Most of these studies have been small and of short duration, and none have had the scientific rigor of the DCCT. However, a systematic review and meta-analysis of these studies done in children and adults has concluded that there are minimal differences between pumps and MDI in A1C outcomes. The combined mean between-group difference favored insulin pump therapy by 0.30% (95% confidence interval −0.58 to −0.02). In addition, there was also little difference in severe hypoglycemia rates in children and adults. In contrast, a report evaluating long-term outcomes of people with type 1 diabetes in Sweden showed a decreased mortality rate from cardiovascular disease in individuals using pumps compared to MDI. For the most part, it comes down to patient preference when deciding between these two treatment approaches.

Studies with Sensors and Sensor-Augmented Pumps

A continuous glucose monitor (CGM) is a device that can give information in real time—glucose values every 5 minutes, arrows indicating the rate of change of glucose values, and alerts and alarms at specific glucose thresholds or predictive thresholds—to help with diabetes management decisions for patients taking either injections or using insulin pumps. The expanded availability and use of CGMs can be partially credited to clinical research results showing the utility of CGMs. With some devices, the pump and CGM are integrated to work together, having the data transferred to and displayed on the pump. This type of therapy is often called "sensor-augmented pump therapy."

The Juvenile Diabetes Research Foundation (JDRF) sponsored one of the largest studies ever done on CGMs. The study included 322 adults and children who were receiving intensive therapy for type 1 diabetes (either with an insulin pump or MDI). After 6 months, adults (>25 years of age) using CGMs showed improved blood glucose control, while participants under 25 years old experienced no improvement in blood glucose control. A subset of children and adults whose A1C values were <7.0% at the beginning of the study was analyzed. In this group of individuals, low blood glucose (hypoglycemia) was less frequent, time spent out of the target blood glucose range was shorter, and average A1C levels were still excellent. The adults and parents of children who used CGMs were also pleased with this method of treatment.

A registry study of over 17,000 participants using CGMs confirmed that more frequent CGM use was associated with lower A1C values. In addition, small randomized controlled trials in adults and children with excellent baseline A1C values (7.0–7.5%) confirmed favorable outcomes (maintaining A1C <7% and reduction in hypoglycemia occurrence) in groups using CGMs, suggesting that CGMs may provide further benefit for individuals with type 1 diabetes who already have excellent glycemic control.

In 2010, the results of the Sensor-Augmented Pump Therapy for A1C Reduction (STAR 3) study were published in *The New England Journal of Medicine*. The STAR 3 study is the largest study of its kind, and it examined the benefits of sensor-augmented pump therapy in people with type 1 diabetes, comparing it against MDI. The study demonstrated that in both children and adults with inadequately controlled type 1 diabetes, sensor-augmented pump therapy improved A1C levels. A1C levels were 0.6% lower than those in the MDI group. Also, a greater number of individuals reached their A1C target levels.

Once the STAR 3 study was completed, the patients using MDI in the first year of the study were placed on sensor-augmented pumps for 6 months. There was a significant and sustained decrease in A1C levels in the children and adults who went from MDI to sensor-augmented pump therapy for the final 6 months of the study.

One of the most important lessons we've learned from all of the clinical studies done with CGM is that the biggest treatment benefit is seen in individuals who use CGMs on a consistent and sustained basis. This is true for anyone on a CGM who wears it continuously, regardless of whether it is used with a pump or MDI. The greatest improvement in glucose control was seen in individuals who wore the CGM for more than 60% of the time, including children, adolescents, and adults.

Since 2010, many other studies have been done in different populations with CGM, including evaluating many studies put together in what is known as a meta-analysis. These studies continue to show the benefit of using CGM in reducing hypoglycemia and, for the most part, in improving A1C.

In 2013, the first large study evaluating an integrated CGM and insulin pump device that automatically stops insulin delivery when sensor glucose drops to a low threshold was published. The threshold-suspend system can stop insulin when sensor glucose drops below a set level between 60 and 90 mg/dL. Once suspended, insulin can be off for a maximum of 2 hours, unless the patient chooses to restart basal insulin at any time up to the 2-hour limit when basal insulin is automatically resumed. The threshold-suspend system was evaluated in 247 patients who were randomly assigned to either sensor-augmented insulin pump therapy with the threshold-suspend feature or standard sensor-augmented insulin pump therapy. The study lasted 3 months, and the main outcomes were nighttime low glucose levels and A1C. The threshold-suspend system was asked to be set to stop insulin delivery at 70 mg/dL. At the end of the 3-month study, changes in A1C values were similar in the two groups, but the threshold-suspend group had a 38% decrease in nighttime low glucose and a 32% decrease in total low glucose events. The percentages of nighttime sensor glucose values of <50, between 51 and 60, and >61–70 mg/dL were significantly reduced in the threshold-suspend group.

In addition to threshold-suspend systems, studies have now been done on systems that have "predictive" low glucose suspend (insulin stops before glucose drops too low), and these systems have also been shown to further decrease low glucose events. Finally, at the time of the writing of this second edition, many studies have been reported evaluating closed-loop systems that have automated insulin delivery. There have been a variety of different systems studied, most for a short time period and in a limited patient population.

These systems are "hybrid," which requires the patient to deliver meal insulin boluses, but then an algorithm in the pump directs insulin delivery automatically, replacing basal insulin. Most of the systems studied use insulin alone in the closed-loop systems, except for a few systems that use both insulin and glucagon (the hormone involved in raising blood glucose).

At the time of the writing of this second edition, only one hybrid closed-loop system has been approved for commercialization. The pivotal study that allowed for device approval was conducted in 124 patients with type 1 diabetes, who were 14 years of age or older. The goal of the study was to assess safety. In addition, A1C and glucose distribution data (to determine the percentage of sensor glucose values below, within, and above 70–180 mg/dL, referred to as the target range) were evaluated before and after using the hybrid closed-loop system. Patients wore sensor-augmented pumps for 2 weeks and then the hybrid closed-loop system for 3 months. During the entire study, there were no episodes of severe hypoglycemia or diabetic ketoacidosis. The average A1C fell from 7.4% at the start of the study to 6.9% by the end of the study. The proportion of in-target sensor glucose values increased, while the percentage in the low and high glucose ranges decreased. Other systems studied in fewer patients and for a lesser time have shown similar improvements in sensor glucose data. And all this is just the beginning.

Guidelines

The American Diabetes Association publishes its guidelines for the management of diabetes every year, with specific mention of special populations, including children. Overall, these guidelines stress the following points:

- Active patient/family participation in pump therapy and continuous glucose monitoring should be strongly encouraged.

- There is no correct age at which to initiate insulin pump therapy or CGMs, so treatment plans should consider the needs of the patient as well as those of the family.

- Robust diabetes education, training, and support is essential for success with all diabetes management, but especially with diabetes technology.

Other medical associations have published recommendations. The International Society for Pediatric and Adolescent Diabetes explains in their guidelines that insulin pump therapy is the best way to imitate how the pancreas in a person without diabetes provides insulin. The American Association of Clinical Endocrinologists has a consensus statement that discusses the broad groups of patients with type 1 and type 2 diabetes who may benefit from insulin pump therapy and the use of CGM.

CHAPTER REVIEW

➡ Appreciate how far you have come since your original diagnosis. You have learned so much about diabetes management, the tasks you need to perform, and ways to better control your glucose levels.

➡ The concepts of basal and bolus insulin delivery are the keys to pump therapy. Both can be adjusted throughout the day and night to improve glucose control. Having CGM data may facilitate meticulous management of glucose levels.

➡ Transitioning from MDI to pump therapy means you go from taking two (or maybe even more) kinds of insulin to one—only rapid-acting insulin.

➡ You should know your blood glucose and A1C targets. You adjust your insulin doses, food intake, and activity levels to reach your glucose targets throughout the day and night. At your diabetes visits, find out your A1C so you can know if you have achieved your goal.

➡ CGM, when used properly, has the ability to reduce A1C, particularly in adults, and may be a useful tool for people with hypoglycemia unawareness or frequent episodes of hypoglycemia. Automation to stop insulin at a preset or predicted low glucose threshold level decreases the risk of hypoglycemia, and now CGM can be used to automate the delivery of insulin, as well.

IN THIS CHAPTER

CHAPTER 2

AN OVERVIEW OF INSULIN PUMPS

WHAT EXACTLY IS AN INSULIN PUMP?

Simply put, an insulin pump is a device that delivers insulin. It is a small mechanical device that is worn externally. It is prescribed by your physician, and your diabetes team will determine your starting doses. You will need to learn how to program the pump, and then you will be responsible for telling it how much insulin to give you. You program it to provide both basal insulin (the background insulin) and bolus insulin (for meals and correction doses). A computer in the pump regulates the flow of insulin into the body. An insulin pump eliminates the use of daily injections and uses only rapid-acting insulin both for the basal rates and for boluses. Wearing a continuous glucose monitor (CGM) with your pump adds benefit in determining insulin doses and in being alerted to aberrations of glucose levels as they are developing. Using a pump with automated insulin delivery is in the early stages, but appears to add benefit, particularly for decreasing low glucose events and A1C, and increasing the time glucose values are in the desired target range.

Durable Pumps and Patch Pumps
Durable insulin pumps are about the size of a deck of cards and can come in a variety of types and colors. Most pumps are connected to the body by tubing. This tubing runs from a reservoir in the pump that you fill with insulin (or in one pump, you can use a prefilled reservoir) to an infusion set. The infusion set is secured to your body with tape. The infusion set is made up of a small 6- to 9-mm (less

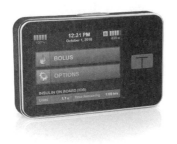
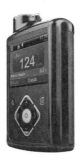
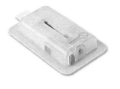

Durable insulin pumps.

than 1/2-inch) soft plastic cannula that is inserted under the skin. It is inserted by a needle, which is then removed. This insertion may be facilitated by a small insertion device. Some of these insertion devices are used over and over again (but only by one person), and others are attached to each infusion set and used only one time. Most infusion sets have a hole or port at the end of the infusion set, but one infusion set also has a side port. The cannula can also be a very small steel needle that is easily inserted under the skin and then left there. The computer in the pump controls a motor that dispenses the insulin in tiny amounts. The insulin flows from the reservoir into the tubing and then through the cannula into the tissue under the skin. There is a display screen on the pump, and there are buttons to program insulin delivery. One pump has the display as a touch screen.

Patch pumps are attached directly to the body. They do not have an infusion set or tubing. The insulin reservoir is inside the small plastic housing on top of the patch adhesive. You fill the reservoir before placing the patch on your body. There is a needle that places a small cannula under the skin, and this needle then retracts back into the plastic housing, so it is no longer in the body. These pumps have a separate controller that communicates with the motor in the patch to control insulin release. There is no display screen on the patch; all interactions are made through the controller, which wire-

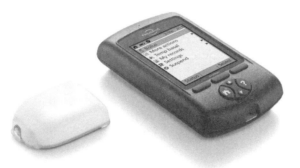

Patch pump.

lessly transmits the commands to the patch pump. There is also a patch pump for type 2 diabetes that is disposable and mechanical. There are preset basal rates that cannot be changed, and boluses are delivered by pressing a button on the patch pump a number of times to deliver the desired bolus dosage. There is no external controller for these.

Those are just the basics. As we go on, you will learn more about what pumps can do, how they work, and what other features pumps have.

ADVANTAGES OF PUMPS

Insulin pumps can be used to effectively manage your diabetes, so let's go over what insulin pumps offer.

Multiple Basal Rates

Multiple basal rates can be used to avoid high and low glucose levels. Many people have specific patterns that can be addressed by changing their basal rates throughout the day and night. A change in basal rate takes about 2 hours to appreciate its effect. For example, if you have the dawn phenomenon (high blood glucose in the morning), then increasing the basal insulin rate at 3:00 A.M. may help you avoid high glucose values that start to increase around 5:00 A.M. If you go to the gym in the afternoon, basal rates can be decreased up to 2 hours beforehand to avoid hypoglycemia. Adjusting rates can also be helpful if you have hypoglycemia unawareness (you don't recognize the signs of low blood glucose), gastroparesis (a digestive disorder), or an unpredictable lifestyle, to mention a few.

Temporary Basal Rates

Pumps allow you to temporarily change basal insulin delivery and to set the amount of time you want this to occur. You can either increase or decrease the basal rate. Decreasing the basal rate helps when you are ill and unable to eat or when you have exercised more than usual and are at risk for hypoglycemia. Increasing the basal rate can help when you have high blood glucose from a variety of factors, such as stress or illness (depending on the illness, the person, whether they can eat or not, and many other factors, glucose levels can go high or low), or when you are particularly sedentary, such as when you are traveling across time zones. In addition, you can use temporary basal rates to help treat highs and lows as they occur. Temporary basal rates can be set by either changing the absolute dosage, e.g., from 0.75 units/hour to 0.7 units/hour, or by using the percent change, e.g., from 100% to 80% of the normal basal rate per hour. Using the percentage change is usually easier than changing the absolute basal rate.

Multiple Basal Patterns

You can have more than one 24-hour basal pattern from which to select. For example, if you are a woman whose insulin sensitivity changes with menstruation, you can program a separate 24-hour basal pattern that increases basal delivery all day long. You can have separate 24-hour basal patterns for weekdays and weekends (when you want to sleep in), for traveling, or for summer vacation. Children may need different basal patterns for the weekdays during school and the weekend if activity levels are different. If you have set multiple patterns, then you just need to be sure you are on the basal pattern you want and that you don't forget which pattern you are using.

Precision in Insulin Delivery

Pumps deliver insulin with precision, particularly when compared with insulin injections. Insulin pumps can deliver very small amounts of insulin, as low as 0.025 units. By contrast, the lowest a syringe can deliver accurately is 0.5 units.

Dosing for Food Intake

Choosing the right dose of insulin for a meal is a huge challenge, particularly if you eat out often, like to snack, or aren't sure what's in your foods. With a pump, you can take multiple boluses by pressing a few buttons, in case you eat more than you planned. You can take one bolus to start with and then take another if you realize the portion you ate was more than you had intended. (Just be careful that you don't take manual boluses.) Even with rapid-acting insulin, dosing at least 10–15 minutes before the meal is optimal, and waiting even longer is important if the glucose value is high before eating. Some people may find giving boluses with a pump is easier and more discreet when you are in public.

Bolus Calculators

Most insulin pumps have bolus calculators that help determine how much insulin is needed for food and for correcting hyperglycemia, and to keep track of insulin-on-board (the amount of insulin you have taken that is still active in your body). By programming your insulin-to-carbohydrate ratio (referred to as carbohydrate ratio, carb ratio, or CR) and correction factor (insulin sensitivity factor, or ISF—how much insulin you need to bring high glucose down to the intended range) into the pump, the bolus calculator will do the math and provide you with an estimate of how much insulin you need to give. Bolus calculators can also be found as apps for cellphones and in blood glucose meters.

Dosing to Correct Hyperglycemia

Because the pump already has your programmed insulin correction factor, it may be easier to take a bolus to correct a high glucose level. Once the glucose level is entered into the pump, the pump will calculate how much insulin is needed. With the push of a few buttons, treatment for hyperglycemia is on the way. But of course, you can still alter that dosage if you feel it is indicated, such as if you know you will be exercising after your meal or snack.

Child Safety Features

Many insulin pumps have features such as button lock options that protect children from accidentally delivering extra insulin or changing pump settings.

Summing Up the Advantages

You can take multiple boluses with the push of a button, have options for basal infusion rates, and get help with insulin dose calculations. And, of course, insulin pumps can be integrated with CGMs and can have automated features.

DISADVANTAGES OF PUMPS

Even though there are advantages to insulin pump therapy, there are also some disadvantages. Understanding them is important, because deciding to go on insulin pump therapy or stay on your insulin pump should be a carefully considered choice.

Risk of Diabetic Ketoacidosis

Because the pump only uses rapid-acting insulin, if there is an unexpected or accidental interruption of insulin delivery, there may not be enough insulin in the bloodstream to stop the liver from releasing glucose and producing ketones. This scenario can rapidly progress to diabetic ketoacidosis (DKA), which is a serious medical condition. By vigilantly monitoring glucose levels, checking the blood or urine ketones, and dosing insulin to bring glucose and ketone levels down, DKA can be avoided. Therefore, it is critically important that you have syringes or rapid-acting insulin pens available for injection, that you never forget how to inject, and that you have devised a plan for management of severe hyperglycemia.

Being Attached

Some people feel apprehensive about wearing an insulin pump all day, every day, and about being attached to a device, no matter how small it is. This apprehension was probably a bigger issue before we all became comfortable having cell phones and exercise monitors with us 24/7. The insulin pump will be attached to you, and for some people, that is a constant reminder that they have diabetes. If it is worn with a CGM, then two things are attached.

Privacy

People can see your insulin pump, unless you conceal it. The pump will make it difficult to hide the fact that you have diabetes if you wish to do so. Even if it is concealed, it may beep or vibrate (and with a CGM, there are more alarms), but these alerts are actually important for maintaining healthy glucose levels.

Skin Issues

The infusion set and the tape can irritate the skin. To use a pump, you may have to try different combinations of tape and skin treatments until you find what works for you. If you use the same site for the infusion set repeatedly, you can get scar tissue and an increase in fatty tissue buildup (called lipohypertrophy). This buildup can also happen if you take injections in the same location every time as well.

Infusion Set Issues

The probability of your infusion set falling out or being jarred from the site can be minimized with good habits. Using appropriate taping techniques and changing your infusion set regularly can help avert problems. To be safe, you need to keep extra pump supplies with you at school or work and have an insulin pen or syringe available so you never have to compromise your safety and health.

Missing Boluses

Some people forget to take a bolus with meals or to correct hyperglycemia. If you regularly miss or skip taking a bolus for food, then your A1C will increase. This increase can happen with multiple daily injections (MDI) as well if you forget a shot. The good news is that many pumps have alarms that you can set to remind you to test or take a bolus at certain times; an example might be to set a bolus alarm to remind you at lunchtime to check your glucose and take your bolus insulin. You can also set the alarm on your phone or watch to remind you about boluses. If you wear a CGM, setting a high alert will also let you know that you might have missed a meal bolus.

Weight Gain

Some people gain weight because of the ease of dosing insulin. But the pump doesn't add excess calories to your meal plan—only you can do that. Remember your meal plan, and schedule a meeting with a registered dietitian if you're having trouble following your healthy eating plan.

Cost

The insulin pump itself plus the supplies (e.g., infusion sets, insulin reservoirs, and tapes) have a cost. Most insurance companies cover insulin pump therapy, minus your deductible. It is important for you to find out what you will have to pay out of pocket for insulin pump therapy before you make the transition. Because the field of diabetes technology is moving rapidly, find out about the pump company's policy for upgrading to new technology as it is developed. Sometimes upgrading through the company may save you more money than going through insurance.

Summing Up the Disadvantages

The disadvantages of pumps include health consequences such as DKA because of a dislodged infusion set or skin issues due to adhesives. The pump will always be attached to you and can be more difficult to keep private with the alarms and alerts. Some people find themselves gaining weight because of the ease of bolusing and allowing themselves to eat more. And finally, insulin pumps can be expensive and insurance may or may not cover their costs. Be sure to think about these topics carefully when choosing an insulin pump.

WHAT MAKES YOU A GOOD PUMP CANDIDATE?

Before anyone can take on an insulin pump, he or she needs to understand what the pump can do and how it works, be realistic about his or her capabilities, and know a good deal about diabetes management. Your diabetes team may be very enthusiastic about pump therapy for you, but are you ready for it? What do you need to do to be considered ready for an insulin pump?

- **Realistic expectations.** The pump doesn't cure diabetes. Pumps with threshold-suspend or predictive-suspend can stop insulin automatically and decrease the occurrence of low glucose levels, and pumps able to dose insulin on their own (with the first of these approved as of the writing of this second edition) have been shown to be safe and able to improve measures of glucose control. Regardless, you must be committed to being very active in your diabetes—and pump—management. Successful management takes time, good habits, dedication, hard work, and commitment.

- **No coercion.** No one should be forced to get an insulin pump, including young children. Although a pump can motivate someone to participate in his or her diabetes management, this cannot be the primary reason to get a child or teen an insulin pump.

- **Participation of others.** No one can manage diabetes alone. Children, teens, young adults, pregnant women, older adults—actually everybody—needs someone who understands diabetes, insulin pumps, and diabetes emergencies. Family members, friends, and colleagues who are supportive and can listen make all the difference.

- **Sufficient diabetes knowledge.** To succeed with pump therapy, it is important to understand the following concepts: basal/bolus therapy and dosage adjustments, your diabetes meal plan, carbohydrate counting, the effects of exercise, how to avoid and treat hyperglycemia, and sick-day management. Gaining skills and knowledge should be your goal. Become a diabetes expert.

- **Awareness of financial responsibilities.** Find out exactly what your insurance will cover and what you will have to pay out of pocket. This is vital information.

- **Sufficient glucose monitoring.** The only way to effectively use an insulin pump is to check your glucose frequently and take action based on the glucose levels. Many health care providers and insurance carriers require proof of four or more glucose checks a day for at least 60 days, or use of a CGM, before they will authorize you to get a pump. Without adequate glucose monitoring, pump therapy is less likely to be successful.

GETTING AN INSULIN PUMP

If you are ready for an insulin pump and are confident that you meet the requirements listed above, then you'll need to work with your diabetes team to determine which pump you should get.

Which Pump?
Different companies make different pumps. Although these different pumps are fundamentally similar, each individual pump has its own distinguishing features and its own relationship with CGM,

DIFFERENCES BETWEEN PUMPS

Lowest basal rate: between 0.025 and 0.5 units/hour

Highest basal rate: between 15 and 35 units/hour

Smallest bolus incremental increase: between 0.025 and 0.01 units

Highest bolus dose: 25–80 units

Time to deliver 1-unit bolus: ~4–40 seconds

Food database: yes or no

Blood glucose meter communication: yes or no

Cartridge/reservoir size: 180–480 units of insulin

Tubing: yes or no

Waterproof: yes or no

and some have automated features. Likewise, different pump manufacturers provide different services. Discuss the available options with your diabetes team, research them on the Internet, read the product brochures, talk to people who use pumps, read the *Diabetes Forecast* consumer guide, and learn as much as possible. Decide what features or services are important to you. Once you have made your choice, work with your diabetes team, the insulin pump company, and a pump trainer to make your new journey successful and enjoyable.

When to Start Pump Therapy

There is no right or wrong time to start insulin pump therapy. It is becoming more common for people to begin pump therapy early in the course of their diabetes, while others wait for some time. Some decide to get an insulin pump only after they have had a problem, like severe hypoglycemia, or a complication. Sometimes the diabetes team is pushing for pump therapy; other times, team members are reluctant. Some health care providers are more willing to use pumps, and others have very strict criteria for who they think is a good candidate.

At the present time, pump therapy is usually considered to be the next step after MDI. In some centers, pump therapy is considered after using a CGM and in other centers, it is considered together with a CGM. It might only take weeks or months to switch to a pump. If your diabetes center starts people on one to three shots per day in a fixed regimen, then you likely have to go to MDI and then to a pump. This could take months or years.

Is there an advantage to starting insulin pump therapy earlier rather than later? Perhaps, but we don't really know for sure. However, data suggest there is no reason to wait until A1C elevates after the honeymoon, or remission phase. More intensive diabetes management is recommended early after diagnosis.

Pump Training

Before you have your in-person pump training, do some research. Most companies have some easy online learning that will help you

IF YOU'RE READY FOR AN INSULIN PUMP, HERE'S WHAT'S NEXT...

Your physician has to prescribe the insulin pump, and your insurance company will have to review and approve the claim. Your pump will be shipped to you or your health care professional. You will be given instructions on how to start learning about your new device.

become familiar with how your pump operates. Your pump trainer will be certified in all of the features of your insulin pump and will verify that you know how to operate it. You will go through all the steps of setting up the pump, filling the reservoir, priming and inserting your infusion set, and practicing as many times as you need until you are comfortable and confident with the pump. There are online tools, instructional videos, and booklets to give you further guidance after training.

Data Management with Computer Programs
You can upload the information stored in your insulin pump, CGM, or glucose meter to a computer program, which is either supplied by the manufacturer of your pump or available from another company. The program will allow you to store and upload information, such as number of insulin doses delivered, pump settings, glucose values, carbohydrates consumed, infusion set changes, pump suspends, device settings, and more. In sensor-augmented pumps, the pump data will be merged with CGM data. These data management programs then display data in pie charts, tables, graphs, and percentages above and below the target range. The ability to transfer these data and analyze them with the software can help you improve your diabetes care by making it easier to detect trends and patterns that may require attention.

CHAPTER REVIEW

➡ An insulin pump is a small machine that continuously delivers insulin. Pumps come in two varieties: durable and patch. Some are combined with a CGM.

➡ The advantages of delivering basal insulin with a pump include multiple basal rates, temporary basal rates, multiple basal patterns, and precise insulin delivery. Boluses can be given at the touch of a button to cover food, to correct an elevated glucose level, or both.

➡ The disadvantages include the risk of diabetic ketoacidosis (DKA), the issues of being attached to a device (or two if combined with a CGM) that remind you about diabetes and the device may be visible to others, issues with your skin and with infusion sets, missed boluses because diabetes management becomes more automatic, and cost.

➡ Pump users should have these qualities: realistic expectations, the ability to participate with others in their diabetes care, sufficient diabetes knowledge, willingness to monitor glucose effectively, the desire to use an insulin pump, and an understanding of and ability to afford the costs of the device.

➡ You need to decide which pump to use, either combined with CGM or not, and perhaps with automated features. Getting properly trained is critical, as is staying motivated.

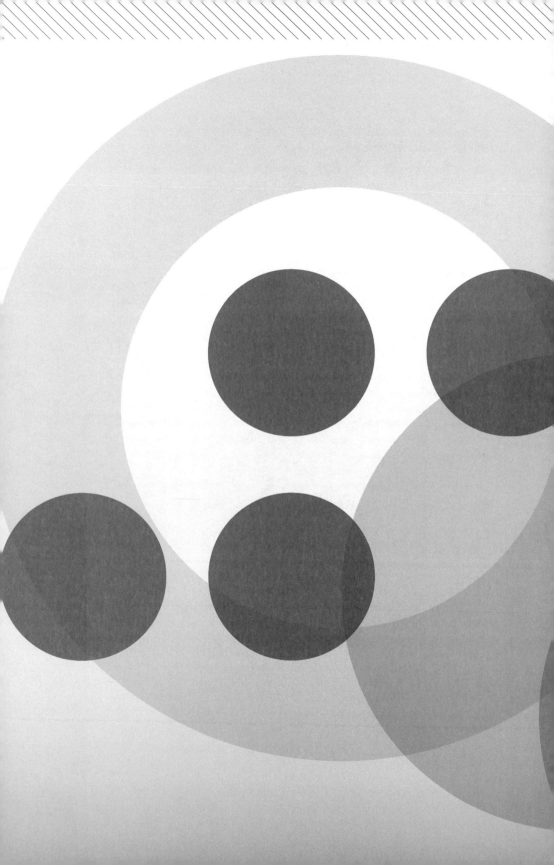

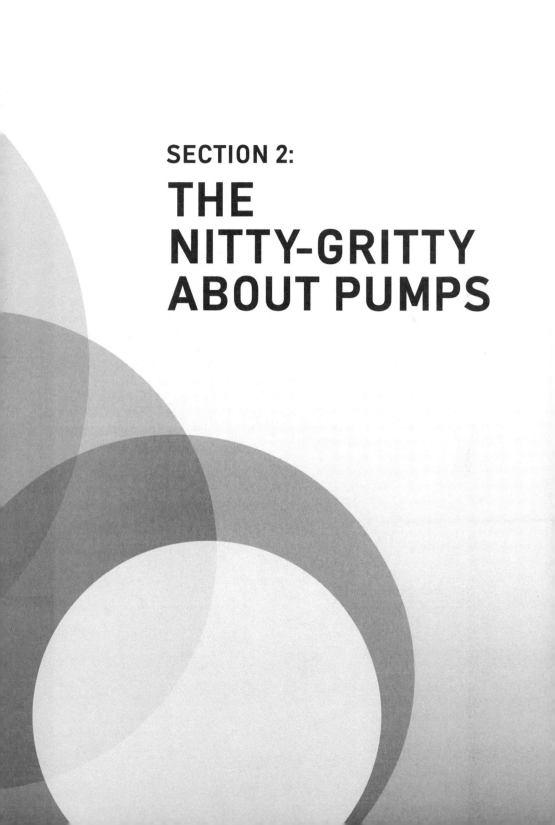

SECTION 2:
THE NITTY-GRITTY ABOUT PUMPS

IN THIS CHAPTER

CHAPTER 3

HOW DOES MY PUMP WORK?

THE PARTS OF THE PUMP

Although only about the size of a deck of cards, an insulin pump is an impressive, complicated device that contains many components and can perform many different functions. There are two kinds of pumps: durable and patch.

Durable pumps are designed to last many years. They are made of a hard plastic case with buttons, a front screen, a battery compartment with a screw-on top, and a space for the reservoir that will be filled with insulin. Clips can be attached to the outer surface so you can place the pump on a belt or waistband. There is a sticker on the pump that has some useful information: the serial number, model and type, company phone numbers, and other general information. At the base of the reservoir shaft is a computer-controlled mechanical plunger that can deliver incredibly small amounts of insulin.

Patch pumps are worn directly on the body. The pod/patch component attaches to the body and has the insulin reservoir and motor inside a small plastic case that is about the size of an egg and about 3/4 of an inch (2 cm) thick. These are disposable. The patch pump is controlled by a separate controller, or personal diabetes manager (PDM). Patch pumps designed for type 2 diabetes are mechanical, have factory-set basal rates, and do not have a PDM. Boluses are delivered by pressing a button on the pump and counting how much insulin has been given.

Reservoir

The reservoir comes empty. There is a needle attachment that is used to draw insulin from the insulin vial into the reservoir. The needle is detached once the correct amount of insulin is drawn up; the correct amount depends on how much insulin you use in 2 or 3 days. The whole reservoir is screw-turned tightly into the chamber in the pump, and the tubing leads away to the infusion set, which is attached to the body. If the pump can use a prefilled insulin cartridge, the cartridge is placed and secured in the reservoir place. With a patch pump, the reservoir is contained within the pod, which adheres to the skin.

Screen

The pump has a front screen that is either controlled by buttons or by touch (the patch pump has the screen on the PDM controller). When not in use, front screens generally display the time (some have the date), insulin remaining, and information about battery life. By pushing different buttons on the face of the pump, you can access different functions in the pump's software. The software lets you deliver insulin; set or edit basal rates; set or edit the pump calculator; suspend insulin delivery; review your bolus, basal, and alarm histories; and see the exact amount of insulin remaining in the reservoir.

Software

The software not only lets you know the date and time, it also allows your pump to store tons of information, including weeks' or months' worth of bolus and alarm histories, blood glucose readings, basal rates, and more. In some pumps, continuous glucose monitor (CGM) data are also stored if it is an integrated system. The software allows the pump to consistently deliver the correct amount of basal insulin. It can also calculate the appropriate amount of insulin needed based on a glucose reading and a carb count entered into the system. Some pumps have a large database of food and carb counts. There are also safety features that prevent the user from providing too much or too little insulin in boluses or for the basal rate. Software also allows you to determine how you want to deliver a bolus every time you deliver one. For young children, there is a lock-out feature for the screen functions.

Pump History and Downloading

The information stored in the pump can be uploaded to a computer and analyzed by software. Generally, the pump connects to the computer using a cable or wireless connection, and once the information is transferred from the pump to a computer, the user can look at graphs, pie charts, lists, and other visual information. Some devices now have advanced analytics and can give information such as events that preceded hypoglycemia and hyperglycemia and patient behaviors. Many diabetes care providers download information from the pump during clinic visits, or they may ask you to download it at home and bring a printed copy to your appointment. Between visits, you should look at this information, try to interpret the data, and send it to your diabetes team if you need help troubleshooting some problems.

Blood and Interstitial Glucose Monitoring

Most pumps can connect to a blood glucose meter. In addition, it is possible for some pumps to connect wirelessly to a CGM. This wireless connection enables the glucose meter and sensor to transmit glucose values directly to the pump's screen and memory. When glucose meters link directly to the pump, it will integrate the glucose level into the bolus calculator for you.

PUMP FUNCTIONS

Insulin Delivery

Pumps deliver basal and bolus rates of insulin to deliver rapid-acting insulin. Basal rates are set by the user, with guidance from the diabetes team. Based on individual dosing, mealtime and correction boluses are given. The temporary basal rate function allows for an increase and a decrease of basal rate to address glucose issues.

Suspend

All pumps have the ability to be suspended so that no insulin (basal or bolus) can be administered. A pump can remain suspended indefinitely but will sound an alarm every so often to remind you that you are not receiving insulin. With most pumps, it is easy to suspend insulin delivery in case you have an emergency, such as impending or actual significant hypoglycemia. Some people also suspend their pumps when they take it off (such as for showers, swimming, or sports) so that no insulin is delivered or wasted when it is not hooked up to you.

Alarms

Pumps have alarms. Some are functionally important, such as "low battery" or "no delivery" (called an "occlusion" alarm in some pumps). There are alarms that you can set to remind you to test, take insulin, or check for ketones if your glucose is over a certain amount. If you need to, you can review the last 50 or so alarms. Pumps have different options for the way they notify you, such as various beeps or sounds or with vibration. Most pumps will beep or vibrate when a bolus is complete, when you are currently using a temporary basal rate, or when you have a low reservoir or low battery. In most pumps, you can choose the alarm volume (or no audible alert), there is a vibrate option available, and you can often turn on or off various types of reminders (for example, missed blood glucose, missed bolus, or low reservoir).

Active Insulin or Insulin-on-Board

After a bolus is given, insulin continues to affect your glucose level for some time. The continued ability of bolus insulin to lower glucose is referred to as "active insulin" or "insulin-on-board." You can set how long you want the pump to track active insulin, but discuss with your health care team how long you should have the pump track it. Generally, people set the active insulin time to 2–5 hours (most often, 3–4 hours). The pump calculator keeps track of the amount of insulin that is still active from previous boluses so you do not have boluses overlapping each other and dropping your glucose levels (this is referred to as "stacking insulin").

Maximal Bolus and Basal Rates

You set a maximal rate for both basal and bolus insulin delivery to enhance safety. This step prohibits you from accidentally taking 20.0 units instead of 2.0 units, for example.

Pump Bolus Calculators Make Pumps Smart

The bolus calculator—which can also be found in pumps, in apps, and on glucose meters—calculates how much insulin to give for boluses. It makes the pump smart and should replace manual boluses. It takes into account your carbohydrate ratio, the correction factor or insulin sensitivity factor (ISF), the duration of active insulin, and your target glucose range. These values (except active insulin) can be altered by time of day, because your insulin sensitivity and your carb ratio may change over the course of 24 hours. When you first get your pump, your diabetes care team will help you determine these settings. They can be changed at any time (preferably in consultation with your diabetes team), as indicated by the patterns in your glucose control. There have been many calculations devised for clinicians when they initiate pump therapy for a patient; these are discussed below.

To determine the amount of insulin you take for a food bolus, you enter the number of grams of carbohydrate you plan to ingest and your current blood glucose level. Most often, you will take this bolus as a surge bolus that gives all the insulin right away (some pumps have slower delivery than others, and some pumps have a way to program whether you want a fast bolus delivery or not). However, depending on the meal quality (high fat, high protein, or very low carbohydrate) or whether you are grazing, you might want to use a dual or square-wave bolus (more about types of boluses in Chapter 5). A dual-wave bolus gives a portion of the total bolus amount taken as a typical, immediate bolus and some portion taken over a longer time period, such as 30 minutes to several hours. A square-wave bolus gives all of the bolus distributed over a longer period of time,

30 minutes to several hours. Then the pump calculator will determine how much insulin you should take. If your blood glucose is above or below your target range, the bolus calculator will also figure out if you need to add or subtract insulin from the food dose.

However, you can always alter the insulin bolus dose suggested by the pump bolus calculator, giving yourself less or more insulin depending on any number of factors. If you are about to exercise or are not sure you will eat an entire meal, you might want to decrease your bolus from what the calculator suggests. If you have ketones or are sick, you might want to take more. Although it is convenient to have the pump calculator so you don't have to do the calculations yourself, it is important to think before you push the button.

Here is an example. If your blood glucose is 250 mg/dL and you are about to eat 15 grams of carbohydrate for lunch, you would enter those numbers into your bolus calculator (or the blood glucose would be automatically sent from your meter). The calculator suggests an amount of insulin to bring your glucose into your target range and cover your meal. Some pumps will show you the two different amounts (one for food and one for correction), and others will simply lump them together into one suggested bolus without showing a breakdown. For these pumps, you can often go to a separate screen with the breakdown of correction and insulin for carbs, before delivering the bolus.

REMEMBER!

Taking your insulin 15–30 minutes before you eat can be an effective way to improve high glucose levels after meals. Before you decide to change your basal rates and/or your carbohydrate ratio, be sure to take your bolus dosage 15–30 minutes before you eat, and determine if that improves your after-meal glucose levels.

UPLOADING AND RECORDKEEPING

Keeping detailed records of your blood and sensor glucose levels, doses of insulin, food intake, and other events (such as exercise, illness, or stress) is important. It is hard to keep a logbook or a record of all that you do every day. However, when this information is available for review, you are able to spot patterns and trends that may be problematic. In contrast, if you are looking only at your current glucose level, you won't detect these patterns, even if you correct your high glucose nearly every morning and treat a low every afternoon.

By uploading data from your pump to the software, especially when it also includes information from your glucose meter (and a CGM, if you have one), you are able to review up to 3 months of data. Because the bolus calculator captures the carbohydrate history for meals and breaks out the bolus details so you can see when correction doses were administered, you have the ability to look for trends and patterns. By reviewing these data, you can identify what the problems are, why they are occurring, and how they can be fixed. This is described in more detail later.

PATCH PUMPS AND PUMPS IN THE FUTURE

Patch pumps have no tubing. The actual computer, with its memory, alarms, history, and bolus calculator, is contained within a separate controller-style device. The controller also contains the blood glucose meter. The "pod" is where the insulin reservoir is filled using a separate needle device. Once the pod is filled, you attach it to your skin with adhesive. Once it is in place, the pod does some automatic checks to make sure everything is working properly and then connects via radio frequency to the controller. After the pod is communicating with the controller, you tell it to insert the cannula. The pod injects the cannula and then retracts the needle automatically. Once the pod is empty, you remove it and throw the whole thing away. Pods last up to 72 hours and then sound an alarm to change the pod. You have 8 more hours after this initial alarm to change the pod before it discontinues and will no longer deliver basal or bolus insulin.

The pods hold a maximum of 200 units and a minimum of 90 units of insulin. If you need 100 units/day, you will need to change the pod every 2 days. On the other hand, if you use <30 units/day, you may find yourself with insulin left in the pod when it expires. If you have 7–12 units left in the pod, this is similar to the amount of insulin left in the tubing of a tubed pump.

Patch pumps at this point do not have the ability to bolus in increments of 0.025 units like some of the tubed pumps on the market. If you have a small child who needs very small increments of insulin, the patch pump at this point may not be the optimal choice, but talking to your health care provider about advantages and disadvantages is important before you decide on a pump.

There is also a pump with a touch screen and a feel that makes it more like a consumer product than a medical one. With all the other essential functions of an insulin pump, the advanced screen has added appeal. There are pumps that hold U500, a type of concentrated insulin, for people who are very insulin resistant as well. But the good news is, innovations in pump design, integration with CGM, and automation of insulin delivery are increasingly available to help you more effectively manage your diabetes.

CHAPTER REVIEW

➡ Understanding the components of the pump, the hardware, and the software, as well as the ability to download and interact with glucose monitors and a CGM, is important.

➡ Make sure you understand basal versus bolus insulin delivery, the pump bolus calculator, the different types of meal boluses determined by the carbohydrate ratio, and correction boluses determined by the insulin sensitivity factor.

➡ The pump has many functions. It has alarms to notify you. It is critical to understand insulin-on-board or active insulin, and the difference between durable and patch pumps.

IN THIS CHAPTER

CHAPTER 4

ALL ABOUT BASAL RATES

WHAT CAN BASAL RATES DO?

One of the great advantages of the insulin pump is that it can be preprogrammed to have one or more basal rates. Basal rates allow for a constant, but variable, amount of insulin to always be present in the blood. This flow of insulin mimics what the pancreas does in people who do not have diabetes; the pancreas always releases some amount of insulin into the bloodstream, but this may vary by time of day.

To remind you, basal rates do the job of long-acting insulin in multiple daily injections (MDI)—that is why basal insulin and basal rates share a name; they do the same job. With MDI, basal insulins cannot be adjusted during the day, whereas basal rates in the pump can be adjusted or fine-tuned throughout the day and night. Pumps use only rapid-acting insulin that is dosed in small, continuous amounts as opposed to long-acting insulin, which is provided only one or two times per day in MDI. If you routinely have physical activity in the afternoon, basal rates can be lowered when insulin requirements are lower. Or if you don't get a lot of physical activity in the morning, then basal rates can be set higher during these hours. Adjustable basal rates also help combat the dawn phenomenon. The dawn phenomenon occurs when certain hormone levels, such as cortisol and growth hormone, spike in the early morning hours, and as a result, blood glucose levels rise and higher amounts of insulin are needed. The advantage of a pump is that it can be programmed to give higher or lower doses of insulin for different parts of the day to more effectively cover activity levels, eating patterns, and other events, like the dawn phenomenon.

Number of Basal Rates

How many different basal rates should you have? This number should be determined by you and your health care team. When you first start on an insulin pump, you may have only one or two rates initially programmed into your pump. However, over the first days or weeks of using an insulin pump, your number of basal rates will likely be adjusted to improve your glucose control. Typically, people end up on two to six basal rates per 24-hour time period.

Adjusting and Suspending Basal Rates

The pump's basal rate can be turned off, decreased, or increased for a period of time to compensate for a sudden, perhaps unexpected, change in glucose levels that results from activity, eating, stress, illness, or other factors. For example, if you plan to exercise for an hour at moderate intensity, but actually end up with 2 hours of high-intensity exercise, then you are at risk for hypoglycemia (because exercise can lower your blood glucose, so the basal insulin rate would send your levels even lower). To protect against hypoglycemia, you could suspend your pump for 30 minutes, decrease the basal insulin delivery by 50% for 1 hour, or use a combination of both. Conversely, if you need more insulin during a sick day, a long car trip, an extended study session, or your period (many teenage girls and young women need more insulin before, during, or after menstruation), then increasing your basal rate can bring your numbers back into the target range.

KEY POINTS ABOUT BASAL RATES

Key points to remember are that it takes about 2 hours to see the effect of a change in basal rate. So if you want to avoid hypoglycemia in the mid-afternoon, you would need to change the basal rate 2 hours before the time you normally go low. And the same holds true for using temporary basal rates.

Determining exactly how long the pump should be suspended or how much basal rates should be increased or decreased takes some practice. It is helpful to keep a log of how and when you alter your basal rates, so you can understand your own pattern.

GOOD TIMES TO CONSIDER SUSPENDING YOUR PUMP
- During and after exercise
- When you have moderate to severe hypoglycemia, particularly at night
- When your glucose level is rapidly falling, to avoid hypoglycemia

Other things to consider:
- Be careful to resume your pump after suspension, because no insulin delivery for more than 2–3 hours may result in ketosis or rebound hyperglycemia.
- Suspending insulin is different than disconnecting the pump; you can disconnect without suspending, in which case the pump continues to give insulin. If you want to eliminate waste of insulin while you are disconnected, suspend your pump. However, effectively disconnecting and suspending insulin do the same thing—keep insulin from entering your body.
- When you take your pump off for a period of time, such as for swimming or bathing, be sure to remember to reconnect after you're done and check blood glucose levels. Correct a high glucose level if necessary.

DETERMINING YOUR BASAL RATE NUMBER AND DOSAGE

Determining the appropriate number and dosage of your basal rates is important. It is important when you first start on an insulin pump, and it is important to know that you and your diabetes team will likely keep changing these over time. This is particularly true in children and teenagers as they grow and go through puberty because children have more variation in their eating and physical activity patterns than adults. So don't be surprised that basal rate adjustments are a routine part of insulin pump therapy. After all, you were always adjusting the dosages of insulin you took when you were on injection therapy.

Total Basal Dosage

How much should your total basal dosage be compared with your total daily dosage (called the total daily insulin dose, or TDD)?

The basal rate typically accounts for between 35% and 50% of a person's TDD. Some people need a greater basal rate percentage (perhaps up to 60%) if they eat a very-low-carbohydrate diet, are very sedentary, or have some other issues. However, some people end up with a higher total basal insulin percentage if they do not take enough boluses of insulin every day—perhaps they forget to routinely bolus for meals (lunch is the most commonly forgotten bolus at school) or don't correct enough for high blood glucose levels. This scenario can result in an increase in basal rates to respond to insufficient bolusing. So, to understand the basal percentage, it must also be compared with the TDD.

BASAL AND BOLUS PERCENTAGES OF THE TOTAL DAILY DOSE OF INSULIN

The STAR 3 (Sensor-Augmented Pump Therapy for A1C Reduction) study (discussed in Chapter 1) showed that adults on an insulin pump with a CGM typically split their TDD between the basal and bolus insulin doses almost equally (<50% basal, >50% bolus). Children and teens on an insulin pump with a CGM used about 35–40% basal and 60–65% bolus in their TDD.

Initial Basal Dosage

Your initial basal dosage is determined by averaging the total amount of all the insulins you use each day for about 1 week. This amount will be a total of your rapid-acting insulin, any intermediate-acting insulin (NPH), and the long-acting or basal insulin. This total is then decreased by about 20–30% because people typically use less insulin when they're on a pump. Then 40–50% of that number becomes the total of all basal rates (some diabetes teams start with even less for the total basal rates). Divide that number, the total of all basal rates, by 24 (for the hours in a day), and you have an hourly rate. Of course, this hourly rate can still be adjusted further depending on any particular patterns or issues.

Another way to calculate the basal dosage is by using body weight. Take your weight in kilograms (your weight in pounds divided by 2.2) and multiply that by 0.7. A 135-pound person would weigh 61.3 kilograms. Multiplying your weight in kilograms by 0.7 will give you the TDD. In this instance, that's about 43 units of insulin a day. After calculating this, determining the hourly rate follows the same process.

Through the process of evaluating and fine-tuning, you will learn when you need more or less basal insulin. You and your diabetes health care team might decide to have two basal rates at the beginning. You might decide to increase the basal rate in the time between 3:00 and 6:00 A.M. to compensate for the dawn phenomenon. Conversely, you may decide to decrease your basal rate in the afternoon, from 3:00 to 5:00 P.M., when you are physically active. Or you might increase the basal rate in the morning because you usually have high glucose levels between breakfast and lunch.

ACCOUNTING FOR BASAL INSULIN THE DAY YOU START THE PUMP

The day you start the pump and start getting basal insulin delivery via the pump, you need to take into account how much basal insulin you have on board from your last basal or long-acting insulin injection. You can take less basal the night before you start pump therapy, or use temporary lower basal rates when you begin using the pump.

CALCULATING BASAL RATES: AN EXAMPLE

Lauren is on MDI, taking 15 units of long-acting insulin in the evening and about 20 units of rapid-acting insulin per day. She's starting on an insulin pump. What would her basal rate be?

1. Calculate TDD.
Add up all of her units of insulin per day.

15 + 20 = 35 (TDD)

2. Calculate insulin pump TDD.
It is common practice to decrease the starting TDD by 20% of what a person was taking with shots, since less insulin is needed when there is greater precision in dosing. Rather than calculating 20% of the TDD and subtracting it, you can simply multiply the TDD by the remaining percentage, which is 80% (100 – 20 = 80%, or 0.80 in decimal).

35 x 0.80 = 28 units

3. Calculate total daily basal dosage.
Lauren will use 40–50% of her TDD for basal insulin. In this example, we'll be conservative and begin with the lowest rate, which is 40%. Multiply her insulin pump TDD by 0.40.

28 x 0.40 = 11.2

Round this down to 11 units of total basal dosage.

4. Calculate the hourly basal rate.
You know how much basal insulin Lauren will need for the day, so we just need to divide that amount by the number of hours in the day to know her hourly rate.

11 ÷ 24 = 0.458

Depending on the insulin pump, you may need to round this rate to 0.45 per hour, since some insulin pumps work in increments of 0.05, while others can work in units of 0.025. The pumps that have working units of 0.025 can deliver basal rates in increments of 0.025, 0.05, 0.075, and 1.0.

Lauren will begin her basal rate at 0.45 units of insulin per hour. She will need to decide with her diabetes team when she will begin her basal pattern so that she does not overlap it with her long-acting basal insulin and cause hypoglycemia. She would probably start her basal rate about 2 hours before she would normally give her evening long-acting insulin, or take less basal the night before if she is starting the pump in the morning, or use a temporary reduced basal rate of 0% or 0.0 units/hour on the pump when she first starts.

HOW TO DO BASAL RATE CHECKS

To understand how to adjust basal rates, you can perform basal rate checks. Checking these rates can be a valuable exercise when you first go on the insulin pump. But doing basal rate checks after you have been on the pump for a while can be even more valuable. In fact, periodic basal rate checks will help you continue to fine-tune your pump settings and maximize your glucose control.

You check your basal rates by avoiding carbohydrate intake during a set period, so you do not have to give a food bolus. Basal rate checks are done when your blood glucose is between 80 and 140 mg/dL or 90 and 150 mg/dL (i.e., your target range, so you don't have to correct a high or low). To see if there is a pattern, you check each basal rate several times. If there is a dramatic dip in your blood glucose while you are checking the first basal rate, change the basal rate to address the low and check that new basal rate.

The first period to be checked is from 10:00 P.M. to 7:00 A.M. You will need to check and log your glucose level every 1–2 hours before you go to bed and then every 3 hours overnight (such as midnight,

---

YOUR INSULIN PUMP SETTINGS

Basal Rates

1. _____ to _____ at units/hour

2. _____ to _____ at units/hour

3. _____ to _____ at units/hour

Bolus Dosages

1. Carbohydrate Ratios (CRs)

1 unit for _____ grams of carbohydrate from _____ to _____ (time)

1 unit for _____ grams of carbohydrate from _____ to _____ (time)

2. Correction Dosages

Insulin Sensitivity Factor

1 unit for every _____ mg/dL out of the target range from_____ to _____ (time)

1 unit for every _____ mg/dL out of the target range from_____ to _____ (time)

3:00 A.M., and 6:00 A.M.). You do this to determine whether you are experiencing overnight lows and highs. Alternatively, use your CGM graph, if you have a CGM.

Next, check your morning rates (7:00 A.M. to noon) so you can see what happens to your glucose level if you occasionally sleep in late, delay or miss breakfast, or have a different schedule for weekends and vacations. During this check, skip breakfast and check and record your glucose every 1–2 hours.

You'll check your afternoon to before-dinner rates next (noon to

BEFORE YOU START BASAL RATE CHECKS...

- You want to check your typical glucose pattern, so avoid situations that affect your glucose levels, like eating, exercise, stress, menstruation, alcohol consumption, and illness.
- Start 4 hours after your last bolus, not any earlier.
- The last meal before you do a basal rate check must have a known amount of carbohydrates so that you can accurately dose yourself for the meal. Prepackaged meals are a good choice.
- Don't do an evaluation if you had a severe low blood glucose earlier in the day.

DURING YOUR BASAL RATE CHECKS...

- Frequent blood glucose checks (every 1–2 hours) are the most important part of these tests! Make sure you check frequently and log all of your results, so that your diabetes care provider can help you determine any rate changes. Or use a CGM.
- If your glucose increases or decreases by more than 30–40 mg/dL during the check, STOP the check and treat the glucose level. If this happens, record it and make sure to tell your doctor.
- Drink water.
- Don't do more than one basal rate check a day.
- Don't stress! This test is to help you fine-tune your care, but if something prevents you from doing a check on the day you originally planned, don't worry. Another day will work, too.

5:00–7:00 P.M., depending on when you eat dinner). Skip lunch and check your glucose every 1–2 hours. Then, to check the dinner to bedtime rate, skip dinner and check glucose every 1–2 hours from 5:00–7:00 P.M. to 10:00 P.M.

If these intervals do not fit your schedule, then you can check for shorter periods or you can divide the overnight, morning, and afternoon periods differently (e.g., 10:00 A.M. to 4:00 P.M. for afternoon).

Don't expect that your basal rates will be perfect. Nothing will work 100% of the time. You are looking for what works most of the time. Look for trends and patterns rather than focusing on specific numbers.

At the beginning of pump therapy, it may not seem easy. Investing more time and effort in the beginning will pay off with less work and better glucose control later. The occasional reevaluation will need to be done for things like daily activity level changes, pregnancy, weight loss or gain, and aging (teenagers often need more insulin during puberty), but for the most part, your basal rates will not change much. Everyday life will seem a little bit easier, and you'll feel better because you're in good control.

Completing basal rate checks like this is great and leads to more precise dosing. But it is also hard to find 3 days when you can skip meals, when you aren't stressed, exercising, having alcohol, sick, or having your menstrual cycle. This is why reviewing downloads frequently can also be extremely helpful. You can adjust basal rates by looking at downloads of a CGM (including a blinded CGM) and glucose levels by looking for patterns in your data. By making small adjustments in response to these patterns, you can effectively address glucose excursions that lead to regular patterns.

IT IS MUCH EASIER WITH A CGM

Because these evaluations require a large number of glucose values, a CGM can be very helpful, including using a blinded CGM if you don't use real-time CGM. If you use a CGM, basal rate checks can be done much easier than with fingersticks.

DIFFERENT TYPES OF BASAL RATES

You can switch between your standard basal pattern and a different preprogrammed basal pattern. Or you can use a temporary basal rate. Basal rates can be temporarily increased or decreased for things like exercise, travel, menstruation, or illness.

Basal Patterns

The basal rates you use for a specific situation are called a "basal pattern" and they cover 24 hours. The basal pattern that you use most of the time is called your "standard pattern." This is the pattern you use most of the time, for your everyday, regular life. But you can preprogram other patterns that you use often, such as sick-day patterns, high patterns, low patterns, weekend patterns, and so on. The names of the patterns in some pumps are listed as "A" and "B," or they can be named by the user. However, regardless of name, they are set up to have a similar kind of function. There are a number of ways to think about these alternative basal patterns. Some people have a pattern that is a 20% increase in (or 120% of) the basal rates in the standard pattern. This pattern is useful for sick days, long travel days with limited activity, or menstruation. Another pattern might be a 20% decrease in (80% of) the standard pattern that can be used for days of high activity or consistent low blood glucose. Some people have a weekday pattern and a weekend pattern. This regime can be useful if you work a very active job and then are more sedentary on the weekends. Any of these patterns can be used for any amount of time, since you can switch back and forth between them as many times as you need. The key to remember is what pattern you are on and to determine if that is the pattern you want.

> The most common rationale for having two patterns: one for weekdays and one for weekends and/or holidays, when you are more (or less) active.

Suspend Basal Insulin Delivery
You can also completely suspend insulin delivery for a period of

time. You might consider suspending basal insulin during exercise, when you have moderate or severe hypoglycemia, or when your glucose level is falling rapidly (confirmed by multiple glucose measurements or a CGM). The pump will indicate that your insulin delivery has been suspended. During a suspend period, it is important to check glucose levels every hour.

Temporary Basal Rates
The other type of basal rate is a temporary basal rate. Temporary basal rates (temp basals) are used for changing basal rate insulin delivery for a fixed period and when you don't want to use a preprogrammed pattern. The temporary basal rate can be set for 24 hours or less. For example, if you are going to go on a long bike ride, you might decrease your normal basal rate by 30% (making your temporary basal rate 70% of the standard pattern) for 3 hours. Once the 3 hours are over, the pump automatically goes to the standard basal rate pattern. In some pumps, the temporary basal rates may be preprogrammed as alternative rates for frequent needs to alter insulin delivery for weekends or nights following exercise.

Temporary basal rates can be changed by units or percentages. For most people, it is easier to use percentage change than unit change. Although small incremental changes can have an effect over time, for impending or actual high or low glucose values, you can consider changing basal rates by a much higher percentage, all the way to 0% or 100%. Using a temporary basal rate of 0 is the same as a suspend. However, a temporary basal rate of 0 can be set for 30 minutes, for example, after which time the pump will automatically restart basal insulin delivery. This tactic is potentially safer than placing your pump on suspend without a time limit in case you fall asleep, or don't hear or pay attention to the "suspend" alarm and forget to resume delivery.

Temporary basal rates can be used when you are running high glucose levels despite taking a correction bolus or boluses (but first be sure the infusion set is not occluded). Increasing basal insulin by 50% or more will help resolve hyperglycemia safely if you turn back to your standard rate once glucose levels start to come down. The same holds true for hypoglycemia, particularly if it is persisting despite glucose ingestion. You can suspend or decrease your basal rate by 75% until glucose starts to increase so that you avoid rebound hyperglycemia.

ADJUSTING YOUR BASAL RATES

When you are ready to start adjusting your basal rates, you should work closely with your health care team. To adjust your basal rates, you need the information from your basal rate checks. Data from your pump will be helpful in understanding recurring glucose patterns.

It is important that changes in your basal rates are made slowly and in small increments. Making dramatic changes to the basal rate can lead to hypoglycemia. For young children, the change in basal rates should be small, such as 0.025–0.05 units per hour; for teens and adults, 0.1–0.2 units per hour will work, but it depends on your own sensitivity factor and how much basal rate you are already getting. Once you make a change, wait 3–6 days (unless you are having lows) before evaluating the results. If you are still experiencing periods of high or low blood glucose, make another small change. However, if you are having frequent, significant lows, it's best to make changes at a faster rate.

Do not try to change several things at once. If you have high morning values and high values before dinner, pick one to remedy. It is usually preferable to work on the overnight and then the morning issues first and then work through the rest of the day in order. Changes earlier in the day may affect later time periods. Studies show that people who have glucose values in range overnight and who wake up with a glucose in range are more likely to be in range during the day as well. Once that change has been made and you no longer are dealing with that issue, start working slowly on the other area. If you are having lows, address those first.

CHAPTER REVIEW

➡ Basal insulin delivery is a key component of insulin pump therapy.

➡ Determining your basal rate dosages is done with formulas. Usually, you start with one or two basal rates and adjust from there. Overall, total basal dosage is 50% or less of your total daily insulin dose (TDD).

➡ Learn how to do basal rate checks, and do them. It may seem complicated when you first start, but assessing how your basal rates are working is very important.

➡ There are different types of basal rates, called basal patterns. You have your standard pattern, which you use most often. However, you might want different basal rate patterns for weekends and weekdays, for when you are running high or low, or for when you travel or have changes in your routine, such as when you are menstruating. Using temporary basal rates can be very helpful, particularly for exercise, stress, and illness.

➡ You should remember that basal rates might change over time. What works now might not work in the future.

CASE STUDIES

SARA

Sara just started a new job and must get up an hour earlier than she had before. When she used to wake up at 6:30 A.M., her morning ritual consisted of a shower and then breakfast at around 7:15 A.M. Now, she must get up at 5:00 A.M., and she eats breakfast at 7:45 A.M. after she gets to the office. She is noticing that her blood sugar levels when she wakes up are in her desired range. However, by the time she gets to work and before she has breakfast, her glucose levels are below her target. She's had hypoglycemia the last couple of days at work, and she's worried that her hypoglycemia will keep her from functioning at her maximum.

Sara wears a CGM and is able to look back at the downloads from her CGM. Her CGM tracings show that Sara's glucose levels start to drop around 6:30–7:00 A.M., and by the time she parks and walks in from the parking garage, she is nearly hypoglycemic.

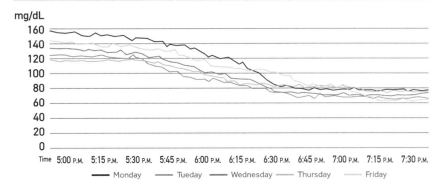

Sara's basal rates are the following: 12:00 A.M., 1.2 units/hour; 5:00 A.M., 1.7 units/hour; 10:00 A.M., 2.0 units/hour; and 5:00 P.M., 1.5 units/hour. Because Sara is experiencing hypoglycemia at around 7:00 A.M., she needs to change her basal rate at least 2 hours beforehand. Sara decides to delay the change in basal from 1.2 units/hour to 1.7 units/hour that occurs at 5:00 A.M. to have the basal rate change occur at 7:00 A.M. Sara understands by waking up earlier and walking from the parking garage to her office, she no longer needs the increase in her basal insulin until later in the morning.

There is no doubt that having CGM data helped Sara make her basal rate change. With a graph of 5-minute glucose levels, it is easy to see where a change needs to be made and that a 2-hour lead time is required. But Sara could have seen the same trend and pattern with blood glucose measurements from her fingersticks. In this case, Sara might need to add one more blood glucose measurement between 6:00 and 6:30 A.M. to assess when her glucose starts to decrease.

CINDY

When Cindy started sixth grade, her health care provider decreased her basal rates because she had a busy schedule in and after school. Despite this, during the first 2 weeks of school, Cindy's mother received four phone calls about afternoon low glucose levels occurring around 2:00 P.M.

Cindy and her mother looked at her pump download and decided to change Cindy's 12:00–2:00 P.M. basal rate from 0.6 units/hour to 0.55 units/hour. After 1 week, Cindy had only one low, during a school challenge to run a mile. Both Cindy and her mother thought this one low did not suggest she needed to change her basal rate again but rather follow her intense exercise plan: take 15 grams of carbohydrate before running, reduce basal rate 50% for 1 hour before and during running and 1 hour after running, and check glucose at midnight and 3:00 A.M.

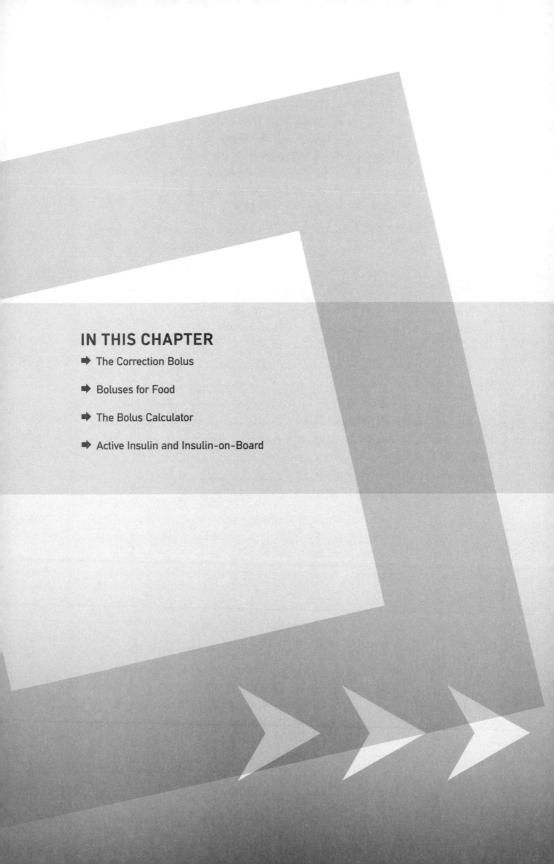

CHAPTER 5

ALL ABOUT BOLUSES

There are two kinds of boluses. A bolus dose of insulin can be delivered to bring a high glucose level back into the target range. This is called a "correction bolus." A bolus can also be delivered to "cover" food (mainly carbohydrate). This is called a "food bolus" or "mealtime bolus." Of your total daily dose (TDD), 50–65% is usually delivered as bolus insulin each day.

THE CORRECTION BOLUS

You want your glucose numbers in the desired range as much of the time as possible. For adults, the American Diabetes Association (ADA) recommends a glucose range of 80–130 mg/dL before meals and <180 mg/dL after meals for many adults, although these numbers should be individualized by the health care team. The more you can keep your glucose in range, the better your A1C levels will be. (Your A1C gives you a 3-month average of your glucose levels.)

This range is most often displayed on CGM screens and data downloads to show you when a glucose number is trending or is too high or too low (these displays may be individualized by changing settings in the device).

The glucose range is different than the target glucose value. The target glucose value is often a single number, like 100 mg/dL, used to determine how much to correct a high or low glucose value. Some pumps allow you to set just a single number (for example, 100 mg/dL), and others allow a range (for example, from 100 to 120 mg/dL).

A correction bolus is given when your glucose is above the upper level of the target glucose value. This target number needs to be set by your diabetes team and is designed to keep your diabetes in good control. The amount of insulin in your correction bolus will change depending on how high your blood glucose level is. If your glucose level is low before a meal, the calculator might subtract insulin from the total recommended amount to account for being below target. Figuring out how many units to take to bring your glucose back to the target glucose value is calculated using your insulin sensitivity factor (ISF).

Insulin Sensitivity Factor

Your ISF determines how many milligrams per deciliter (mg/dL) 1 unit of insulin will decrease your glucose level. For example, if 1 unit of insulin is expected to bring your glucose down by 50 mg/dL, your ISF would be written as 50. You may already be familiar with your ISF from multiple daily injections (MDI) therapy.

Using Your ISF to Correct Blood Glucose Levels

Use your target glucose value to figure out how many units of insulin it will take to bring your glucose back into your range. If your target range is 80–120 mg/dL, for example, find a number in the middle of this range, such as 100 mg/dL, to use as a target number for your calculations. For practice, pretend you just tested and your glucose is 200 mg/dL and your ISF is 50. You can calculate your units of correction insulin by subtracting your target glucose (in this case, 100 mg/dL) from your current blood glucose (in this case, 200 mg/dL). Then you divide your answer by your ISF to figure out how much insulin you need to get back to your target of 100 mg/dL.

The equation for a blood glucose reading of 200 mg/dL, target of 100 mg/dL, and an ISF of 50 would look like this:

$$200 - 100 = 100$$
$$100 \div 50 = 2$$
Total correction bolus = 2 units

Calculating Your ISF

You're probably wondering how you find out your ISF in the first place. Your diabetes team will help you calculate your first ISF when you're starting on insulin pump therapy. But you can also calculate it yourself. The process starts with the 1500 Rule, the 1700 Rule, or the 2000 Rule. The 1500 Rule is for people who have insulin resistance or require more insulin; the 1700 Rule is for people who have a standard insulin response; and the 2000 Rule is for adults or children who are insulin sensitive and require less insulin. After choosing a rule and applying it, you can adjust from there to get the desired effect from your correction dosage.

In this example, we will use the 1700 Rule. Start by dividing 1700 by the TDD you use for your pump. Your TDD is 34 units.

$$1700 \div 34 = 50$$

This means that you will need approximately 1 unit of insulin to bring your blood glucose down 50 mg/dL, which would make your ISF 50 (if you get a number that is not whole, just round to the nearest whole number). As with all starting doses that are based on formulas, you will need to closely monitor your glucose levels and perform specific checks to fine-tune the initial settings.

ISFs are not stagnant; they can change over time. They may need to be adjusted when you get older, change activity levels, or go through puberty, as well as during different hours in the day. The way to know whether your ISF is correct is to be aware of how your body reacts to your correction doses and to notice patterns of highs or lows. Many people notice that they are less sensitive (or more resistant) to insulin in the morning (during the dawn phenomenon), so they will need more insulin in the morning than in the afternoon or evening. For example, the morning ISF might be 40, compared with 50 for the afternoon and evening. It is important to understand that "less sensitive" means 1 unit of insulin will bring you down a lower number of milligrams per deciliter (mg/dL) in the glucose level; thus, it will take more units of insulin to get you into the desired range. The less sensitive factor of 40 means that to come from 250 to 100 mg/dL, you will need 3.8 units of insulin. "More sensitive" means

1 unit of insulin will bring you down a greater amount in the glucose level. The more sensitive factor of 50 means that to come from 250 to 100 mg/dL, you will need 3.0 units of insulin.

Some people have two or even three ISFs for a 24-hour period. Insulin pumps will remember your different ISFs and use them in your pump bolus calculator at the appropriate times.

Checking and Evaluating Your ISF

As with the evaluation of basal rates, you need to verify that your ISFs are right for you. You accomplish this by checking them. You do ISF checks after you have corrected a high glucose level and when you can see how the correction bolus brings your glucose level down without other factors affecting it. You can do an ISF check when you have not eaten carbohydrates for 3–4 hours and don't have any active insulin from a previous food bolus. You also do ISF checks when you have not exercised, been ill, or been stressed for at least 3–4 hours (or had alcohol for 24 hours). It is important that you know your basal rates during this time are accurate. If they are too high or low, then you may be compensating in your ISF.

When you find that it has been 3–4 hours since your last meal and your glucose is elevated out of the target range, you can do an ISF check. Give your correction bolus, and check your glucose levels every 1–2 hours after the initial correction bolus. Record your results.

If 3–4 hours have passed since your correction bolus and you are not back in your target range, you might consider repeating this procedure on another day. If you have the same results on a second test, you might want to consider changing your ISF in the pump settings.

Examples

If your ISF is 43 and your glucose is 250 mg/dL, you would take 3.5 units to bring your glucose to 100 mg/dL (250 − 100 = 150; 150 ÷ 43 = 3.48, rounded to 3.5). If your glucose was 167 mg/dL at 4 hours during your ISF check, then you need to change the factor, because the correction bolus has not sufficiently lowered your blood glucose. You could try 40, so you'd need 3.75 units (150 ÷ 40 = 3.75). You lower your ISF because you need more insulin to lower your blood glucose to the desired level. You could also try an ISF of 37, which would mean that you would have taken 4.05 units to correct (150 ÷ 37 = 4.05).

Conversely, if your blood glucose is lower than target at any point during your ISF check, you may need to change your ISF in the opposite direction. In this case, you might want to change from 50 to 70. Therefore, you would have taken 2.1 units for this correction (150 ÷ 70 = 2.14, rounded to 2.1). You need less insulin to bring your glucose to the target.

BOLUSES FOR FOOD

Insulin boluses regulate glucose levels in response to the food and drink you consume, especially when they contain carbohydrate (sometimes called carbs, or written as CHO). Carbohydrates are broken down into sugar molecules, which are used as fuel by your cells. Insulin allows this sugar to enter into the cells and to be used for energy. Because a person with diabetes does not have enough insulin in his or her body or because the body is more resistant to the effects of insulin, insulin injections or boluses must be used to replace insulin. These mealtime doses of insulin are called meal or prandial boluses, and this kind of bolus is given as an injection (on MDI) or by the push of buttons on an insulin pump.

Carbohydrate Ratio (CR)

The bolus calculator in the insulin pump can calculate the amount of insulin needed for the amount of carbohydrate ingested. This uses your "carbohydrate (carb) ratio," or CR. You might already have had a CR from when you were on MDI therapy. These CRs might change in response to being on an insulin pump. It is a good idea to recalculate and reevaluate your CRs. If you didn't have a CR(s), you have to calculate one by reading below.

Calculating Your CR

To determine your CR, most people use the 450 Rule. The 450 Rule is similar to the 1700 or the 2000 Rule for determining ISF.

You divide 450 by your insulin TDD. Let's use the same example we used for calculating ISF, when the TDD was 34. If your TDD is 34, then 450 ÷ 34 = 14.7 (you can round to the nearest whole number if needed, in this case to 15), so 1 unit of insulin is needed for every 15 grams of carbohydrate ingested. The CR equals 15.

Some people might have several CRs throughout the day. Most people have a different CR at breakfast than for the rest of the day because insulin sensitivity is often decreased in the morning due to a natural influx of hormones when you wake up. Therefore, more insulin is required per gram of carbohydrate than for meals later in the day. For example, a CR at breakfast may be 12, whereas it may be 15 during the rest of the day.

Checking and Evaluating Your CR

You can check whether your CR is correct, just like you can check your basal rates and your ISF. You accomplish this by doing CR checks. You can check your CR when you have a glucose reading before eating that is in the target range and when you can accurately calculate the amount of carbohydrate you are ingesting (in food and beverages). This step gives you the ability to see how the CR works for your food and beverages without other factors affecting it. For example, make sure to do CR checks when you have not had to correct a high glucose value for 3–4 hours and when you don't have bolus insulin that is still active from previous food boluses or correction doses. Also, do CR checks when you have not exercised, been ill, or been stressed for at least 3–4 hours (or had alcohol for 24 hours), just like when you check your ISF.

After the food bolus (determined by the bolus calculator) is given, check your glucose every hour for 4 hours, or watch your CGM tracings. The ADA recommends that postmeal blood glucose levels in adults be no higher than 180 mg/dL after meals, typically 1–2 hours after eating. If, during the 4 hours after eating (without more food or exercise), your glucose reading is back in the target range (<180 mg/dL), then the CR is correct. If, after 3–4 hours, your blood glucose is above the target range, then the CR should be changed to give more insulin per gram of carbohydrate. This is referred to as "lowering your CR." If your glucose is below the target, then your CR should be changed to give less insulin per gram of carbohydrate, "raising your CR." CR is similar to ISF with how lowering the number increases the amount of insulin you get for a specific amount of carbs. If you have a 15 CR and your glucose is higher than your target 4 hours later, you need more insulin, so you lower the number in your ratio. You could reduce your 15 to 12 and see if the 4-hour glucose level is in range.

There is one other thing to think about with boluses: if at 4 hours your blood glucose is in the target range, but there were values higher than 180 mg/dL within that 4 hours, you might need to think about the timing of your insulin bolus for food. Taking your insulin 15–30 minutes before you begin eating improves your control.

Here are two examples. If your CR is 15 and you ingest 60 grams of carbohydrate for lunch, then you'll take 4 units of insulin to cover the meal (60 ÷ 15 = 4). If at 4 hours your glucose is 225 mg/dL, then you need to decrease your CR. You can try a new CR of 12. You would then take 5 units of insulin for a 60-gram carbohydrate meal (60 ÷ 12 = 5). This is because you need more insulin to keep your glucose level in the target range after eating. If you tried a new CR of 10, then you would take 6 units of insulin (60 ÷ 10 = 6).

Don't forget that when you make a change to your CR, ISF, or basal rates, you should only change by about 10–20%.

Conversely, if your glucose is lower than target at any point within 4 hours after your meal, you may need to increase your CR. You might want to change from 15 to 18. In that case, you would have taken 3.3 units (60 ÷ 18 = 3.33). You need less insulin to cover your meal.

Timing the Food Bolus

In general, it is best to give the insulin bolus 15–30 minutes before eating. It takes about 15 minutes for carbohydrate to start to influence your blood glucose levels, with peak effects around 60 minutes after eating. Even rapid-acting insulin takes longer to start working, reaching its peak effect at 90–100 minutes after a bolus.

With young children, it is often difficult to determine how much they will eat. It has been shown that giving insulin after the meal can still allow for good diabetes control. If you do this, and the young child decides to eat less, you will not have given them too much insulin. However, for the most part, it is better to give a little insulin before eating and then play "catch up" as food is consumed. For example, if a young child usually eats 22 grams of carbohydrate for breakfast and has a CR of 20, then you can guess that the child will probably need 1.1 units of insulin (22 ÷ 20 = 1.1). You can give a fraction of this dose before the meal, such as 0.2–0.4 units, and then give the rest as the child is eating or when the meal is completed. One major advantage of an insulin pump is, it is easy to give some insulin before the meal if you are not comfortable giving the full dose in advance.

Bolusing for Carbohydrates and Correction

When you are ready to eat a meal or snack or drink something with carbohydrate, you should check your glucose before you start eating or drinking and count the carbohydrates you're going to consume. Your glucose before you eat or drink will be within your target range, above your target range, or below your target range. Check your glucose with a fingerstick or CGM. Recently, the U.S. Food and Drug Administration (FDA) approved the use of CGM values from one commercial product in the U.S. for bolus dosing of food and correction, instead of doing a confirmatory fingerstick blood glucose measurement. The hybrid closed-loop system has approval for basal insulin dosing through the algorithm based on CGM values. However, not all CGM systems have FDA approval for insulin dosing at the time of this second edition. Check with your CGM company to determine what is approved.

Within Target Range

If your glucose is in the target range, then you take insulin to cover the carbohydrate.

Above Target Range

If your glucose is higher than your target, you have two choices. You can correct the elevated glucose first and wait 30 minutes or more until your glucose comes back into the target range. Or you can take a bolus that adds the correction dose of insulin to the dose you are going to take to cover your carbohydrates. If you do this, you should wait 15–30 minutes (or even longer if the glucose is very elevated) after the bolus before you start eating to allow your glucose level to start to come down first. A method some people use to determine how long to wait before eating is to use the first two values of the glucose level as minutes before eating. If the glucose is 287 mg/dL, they will wait 28 minutes from the time of the bolus to the time they start to eat.

Below Target Range

If your glucose level is below target before you start to eat—in the hypoglycemic range—what should you do? There are a few options:

- Consume 15 grams of carbohydrate to correct your glucose level before you eat (if your child is younger than 10 years of age, you might want to give only 8 grams) and wait 15 minutes. Check your glucose. If it is still low, consume another 15 grams of carbohydrate and check again 15 minutes later. Repeat this process until you are back in the target range. This is called the "Rule of 15s," because you eat 15 grams and you wait 15 minutes. Once your glucose is back in the target range, you can take your insulin dose to cover the carbohydrate in your meal. This is particularly helpful if you were going to eat a high-fat meal, because a lot of fat will slow the effects of carbohydrate on your blood glucose levels.

- Decrease your insulin bolus using the pump's bolus calculator. For example, if your target range is 90–100 mg/dL and your glucose is 70 mg/dL before you plan to eat a 45-gram carbohydrate meal, you can use the bolus calculator's settings to estimate a dose that subtracts some insulin, taking into account that your glucose is a little low.

- Decrease your insulin bolus by considering some of the carbohydrate you are about to eat as "free" (meaning that it will not be treated with insulin). So if your CR is 15, you would normally take 3 units of insulin for a 45-gram carbohydrate meal. For example, if your premeal glucose is 60 mg/dL, it is recommended that you ingest 15 grams of carbohydrate as "free." So you subtract 15 from 45, and use only 30 grams of the carbohydrate that you are going to eat in calculating your meal bolus. This means you would only take 2 units of insulin for the meal. You might even consider waiting until after you have started eating and the food has begun to elevate your glucose level before taking the full bolus. Talk to your diabetes team about which option may be best for you and have a plan for what to do before you actually have hypoglycemia.

Bolus Types

There are different types of food boluses. These different boluses can extend the time over which the bolus is delivered by your pump.

Regular Bolus

A regular bolus delivers all of the insulin over a short period of time. The amount of time it takes depends on how fast the pump motor can give the dose. This is generally less than 5 minutes in duration.

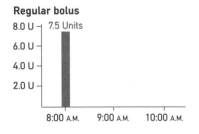

Square-Wave or Extended Bolus

A square-wave (or extended) bolus dispenses insulin over a specified amount of time. This is good for high-fat meals because the stomach empties more slowly after a high-fat meal, and a regular bolus of insulin might cause blood glucose levels to go low. This bolus can also be used for long periods of snacking (such as at parties, sporting events, and movies).

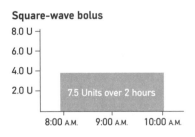

Dual-Wave or Combination-Wave Bolus

A dual-wave bolus is a combination of a regular meal bolus, which is given all at once, and the square-wave bolus. This combination is good for high-carb/high-fat meals, like pizza and Chinese or Italian food. Generally, the total calculated bolus is given as 50% in a regular food bolus and 50% in the square-wave bolus. For example, if a 7.5-unit bolus is calculated for a meal, then 4.0 units will be given at the beginning and 4.0 units will be spread out over a certain amount of time (normally 2 hours). These figures will vary depending on the individual. Different types of meals might also require different distributions of the bolus (for example, pizza versus Chinese food). Over time, you will figure out which combination works best for you.

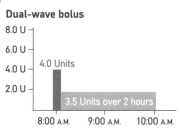

Dual-wave bolus

4.0 Units

3.5 Units over 2 hours

8:00 A.M.   9:00 A.M.   10:00 A.M.

THE BOLUS CALCULATOR

Pumps have bolus calculators that make it easier and safer to give more accurate doses. The bolus calculator uses personalized settings that are prescribed by your diabetes team, keeps track of your previous boluses, and does the complicated math to provide an estimated dose. The bolus calculator will provide a suggested

TAKE ADVANTAGE!

Take advantage of your pump's ability to do square-wave or dual-wave boluses. It can be extremely helpful to use these functions. The only way to really know which bolus type will work best for your body and the food you eat is to try these boluses and monitor your blood glucose 2 and 4 hours after your meal. Many people will start with a 2- or 3-hour period of extended delivery. In the case of the dual-wave, take half the needed insulin as a regular bolus and half over an extended period of time. People who use these different bolus methods might find that their blood glucose levels are better managed.

BOLUS CALCULATOR SETTINGS AND INFORMATION

Bolus calculator settings that are programmed into the pump during setup (these may vary at different times of the day and night) include the following:

- Glucose target range
- CR
- ISF
- Active insulin time

➡ Your current glucose level is either entered by you or transmitted automatically from your glucose meter.

➡ You enter the number of grams of carbohydrate that you plan to eat each time you give a bolus for food.

dose. It is your responsibility to take into consideration other important factors that could be affecting your insulin requirements (such as exercise or illness) and to decide whether you are going to deliver the suggested dose or adjust the estimate before delivering the dose.

If you have a CGM, use this to watch how glucose levels respond, and review downloads to check your different ratios. You can get a good idea of how glucose levels respond to your bolus doses each day.

ACTIVE INSULIN OR INSULIN-ON-BOARD

When you are calculating a correction bolus for a high glucose value, you may still have bolus insulin in your system from a previous food or correction bolus. The amount of insulin left in your bloodstream is referred to as active insulin or insulin-on-board (IOB). The amount of active insulin or IOB decreases as time passes because your body absorbs the insulin in the bloodstream. Your insulin pump can calculate the remaining active insulin using the active insulin or IOB setting. It is important to consider the presence of active insulin or IOB, because taking a correction bolus on top of active insulin (known as "stacking insulin") can lead to hypoglycemia.

For example, if you ate a big meal and took a bolus 15 minutes before eating, you may still have an elevated glucose level 2 hours later. If you want to correct this after-meal high, you should not take a full correction dose. You should account for the active insulin or IOB that is still in your blood from your meal bolus. If you plan on eating more carbohydrate, you might want to only dispense a bolus for the extra carbs you are going to eat and not add any correction at all. Or you can add a correction dose that is modified by the active insulin or IOB. If you choose to give a full correction bolus and a food bolus when you have active insulin in your system 2 hours after your previous bolus, then you would be stacking insulin and increasing the chances that you'll go low. Pump bolus calculators reduce correction doses by deducting IOB from the initial calculation. Some pumps use either a linear or curvilinear action profile to calculate IOB. All boluses, food and correction, are reduced by IOB in some pumps, while other pumps only reduce correction boluses.

The concept of active insulin or IOB also applies to correction boluses. If you corrected at noon but your glucose level was higher 1 hour later, then you would not want to take a full correction bolus for this new higher glucose level because you still have IOB. Instead, you would take a decreased bolus that accounts for how much active insulin is still in your blood from the first correction bolus.

The pump bolus calculator will calculate all these different factors together when you enter your blood glucose and the number of carbohydrates you plan to eat. The pump stores all of your ratios and factors for use in these calculations and will also incorporate active insulin or IOB. The calculator will suggest a dose, but you are always able to make changes to it (in the event of increased activity, for example).

However, always be sure to check for ketones in situations in which the risk of diabetic ketoacidosis (DKA) is present. Pump calculators do not calculate the extra insulin that is needed when someone has ketones (see Chapter 13).

Conditions that can increase your glucose levels:	Conditions that can decrease your glucose:
Anxiety/stress	Exercise
Fatty foods/high-protein foods	Weight loss
Caffeine	Aging
Growth and weight gain	Alcohol
Inactivity	High altitude, heat, humidity
Rebounding from a low glucose	Vomiting, gastrointestinal illness
Some medications	Some medications
Illness/surgery	Mental activity
Menstruation	Menstruation

CHAPTER REVIEW

➡ Bolusing the right amount at the right time and for the right reasons is a key to success. Correction boluses help manage diabetes and depend on obtaining the right ISF. You calculate your ISF with specific formulas, and these may vary throughout the day. Do correction bolus checks to be sure you have the right ISF to bring you back to the target range after a high glucose level and without increasing hypoglycemia.

➡ Food boluses are calculated with formulas, and these may change throughout the day and night. Many people need more insulin for carbohydrate in the morning. You should check and evaluate your CR to be sure you have the right CR to manage your diabetes. You need to understand the importance of the timing of food boluses, correctly counting carbohydrate, and determining which bolus—normal, square-wave, or dual-wave—to use.

➡ The bolus calculator provides a huge advantage in insulin pump therapy by helping to determine how much insulin is needed for food and correction boluses.

➡ The bolus calculator also considers active insulin, or insulin-on-board (IOB), to ensure that safe boluses are delivered. This step helps prevent insulin stacking and the resulting hypoglycemia.

CASE STUDY:
DETERMINING HOW TO USE
THE EXTENDED BOLUS FEATURES

ROB

Last football season, Rob and his neighbor watched the Sunday afternoon game together. Rob would make a pot of chili and sourdough rolls, and they would slowly eat lunch while they jumped up and down watching the game. At the beginning of the season, Rob realized that even when he calculated his carbs by measuring the chili and eating half a roll, he would have an immediate postmeal dip in his glucose, and then his glucose levels would run high all evening.

Rob decided to calculate not only the carbohydrate content of what he was eating but also the protein and fat. For chili, he ate 1.5 cups with 2 oz of shredded cheese on top, for a total of 25 grams of carbs, 17 grams of protein, and 18 grams of fat. Half of the sourdough roll was 21 grams of carb, 4 grams of protein, and 1 gram of fat. His CR was 5, so he would normally take 9.2 units for lunch.

Because of the unwanted glucose pattern that Rob initially experienced, he made an appointment with his dietitian. They discussed the value of using a dual-wave bolus because he was eating over about 1.5–2 hours and because of the high fat content of the meal. Rob took half (4.6 units) as an immediate bolus and then the remainder as an extended square-wave bolus over 3 hours. When he tested his blood glucose 2 hours after eating, as well as before going to bed, he was in his target range. The dual-bolus enabled him to eat slowly and to also compensate for the high-fat quantity of his Sunday afternoon football-watching meal.

IN THIS CHAPTER

CHAPTER 6

UNDERSTANDING THE MEAL PLAN

A healthy, balanced nutrition plan is the key to strong diabetes management. It is important to understand how the foods and beverages you eat and drink affect your glucose levels. It is just as important to understand how much insulin you need to take for what you eat and drink. Carbohydrate is the main nutrient that affects your glucose levels, so you need to learn how to count carbohydrate. But you must also understand how the other macronutrients—fat and protein—interact with carbohydrate to customize your insulin use to your body's individual needs. These are critical skills to have in your journey with diabetes.

FIXED MEAL PLANS

Before the discovery of insulin, the only thing that could be done to help someone with type 1 diabetes survive was to restrict his or her intake of carbohydrates and calories. After the discovery of insulin, people were put on a fixed dietary plan. They were not allowed to have simple carbohydrates (sugars). They were told they needed to eat the same thing—mainly protein, complex carbohydrates, and fat—at the same time every day so that glucose peaks from food could be matched by insulin peaks from one, two, or three injections a day. As a result, people were forced to eat at set times whether they were hungry or not and were not allowed to eat at other times, even if they were hungry. If they ate more or ate during these forbidden times, they were accused of "cheating." The diet was difficult and dreary, and following it was not fun for most people with diabetes.

The Exchange Diet

The original fixed diet plan evolved over time into a number of different nutrition plans. One of the most popular plans was called the Exchange diet. The Exchange diet was based on breaking down the components of the diet into "exchanges." In this way, you could exchange one food for another, provided they both contained a similar amount of nutrients and calories, thereby allowing the diet to be more varied. For example, a carbohydrate could be exchanged for a different carbohydrate of equal quantity, one protein could be exchanged for another protein, and fat could be exchanged for fat. Because carbohydrate management is essential in diabetes, the exchange system focused on carbohydrates. Various carbohydrates were compared to a slice of bread (or 15 grams of carbohydrate), and this was known as one carbohydrate exchange or one "carb choice." An apple, half a banana, a half cup of pasta, and half a baked potato were all one carbohydrate exchange. With the Exchange system, the number of exchanges (or choices) that you were allotted per meal was dictated by your dietitian or health care provider. The Exchange system is no longer the preferred nutrition plan for someone with type 1 diabetes (carb counting is), but its principles are used in some weight-management programs because this method highlights nutritional composition and serving size.

In 1995, a few years after the Diabetes Control and Complications Trial (DCCT) results were reported and the importance of intensive diabetes management was realized, the Exchange system underwent revision and improvement. It began to be based more on counting carbohydrates. You were no longer obligated to eat carbohydrate in 15-gram portions or in amounts equivalent to an exchange. Instead, you count individual grams of carbohydrate and link grams of carbohydrate with units of insulin, via the carbohydrate ratio (CR). Once rapid-acting insulin came onto the scene, the world was ready to switch directly to carb counting.

Regardless of the type of meal plan that you follow, it is important to space your meals and snacks so there is at least 3 hours between for your glucose level to come back to (or close to) premeal levels. Eating all the time, which some people refer to as grazing, usual doesn't allow optimal glucose control.

ALL ABOUT CARBS

Carbohydrates are sources of energy—fuel for our bodies. Your gastrointestinal tract breaks down carbohydrate into individual sugar molecules. This group includes starches (bread, pasta, potatoes, cake, etc.), disaccharides (lactose, maltose, and sucrose), and simple sugars (glucose, galactose, and fructose). Fiber, like that found in vegetables, is also a carbohydrate.

Types of Carbohydrate

There are three types of carbohydrate, and all affect your blood glucose levels. Starches (complex carbohydrate), sugars (simple carbohydrate), and fiber are all forms of carbohydrate. Starch and sugar cause blood glucose levels to spike and generally have a higher glycemic index (covered later in this chapter). Foods high in complex carbohydrate (i.e., starches) include vegetables, such as potatoes, corn, and winter squash, but also include grains, pasta, breads, cereals, cookies, cakes, and more. Simple sugar and sucrose are broken down and enter the blood quickly and are found in foods like honey, milk, syrup, table sugar, fruit, and fruit juices.

Each gram of starch or sugar counts as a gram of carbohydrate. So, if you eat a small apple, it has 15 grams of carbohydrate. Generally, a small piece of bread has 15 grams, as does one serving of pasta (1/2 cup). A serving of cereal might be anywhere from 15 to 45 grams, depending on the portion size.

Fiber, even though it is a carbohydrate, is a bit different. Your body can't break down all fiber. Therefore, fiber is never fully converted to glucose. If a large portion of the total carbohydrate in your meal comes from fiber (generally about 5 or more grams of fiber), you can reduce the number of carbs you're counting in your meal by the amount of fiber. For example, if you eat 36 grams of carbs and 7 grams of that is fiber, then you would use 29 grams of carbs to calculate your meal bolus (36 − 7 = 29). Fiber is the reason you often hear some vegetables referred to as "free foods." A "free food" is a vegetable you can eat and not have to take insulin. This doesn't mean that broccoli doesn't have carbs; it does. Broccoli doesn't have many carbs, and about half of those carbs are as fiber. One cup of raw broccoli has about 6 carbs, but 2.5 are fiber. For most people with a CR of 10–15, they would have to eat a lot of broccoli to need to take insulin for it.

There is evidence that when you are on an insulin pump, it is best to manage your diabetes by using carbohydrate counting (usually shortened to "carb counting" or "counting carbs"). By counting carbs, you know how much insulin to dose. This process is made easier because food labels are required by law to show you how much carbohydrate is in each serving of food. Reading the food label (which is covered later in this chapter) is important and makes diabetes management easier. With the help of the food label, you can determine the amount of carbohydrate per serving size of the food. When used with your CR, you can successfully determine how much insulin is needed to cover a meal. Carb counting, your CR, and your pump combine to be a powerful toolbox for managing your diabetes.

Carb Counting
The more accurate you are with your carb counting, the better your diabetes management will be when you use insulin pump therapy.

FOR YOUR REFERENCE
An excellent guide to the skills of carb counting is the *Complete Guide to Carb Counting*, 3rd edition, by Hope S. Warshaw and Karmeen Kulkarni, published by the American Diabetes Association.

Thankfully, once you know how to read a food label, understand how to measure your portions (with scales, measuring cups, serving spoons, etc.), and can calculate your CR, determining how much insulin to dose can be a rather straightforward practice. You will need to work with your diabetes team, especially a registered dietitian, to become skilled at carb counting. You will need to learn about basic nutrition and read some carb-counting books so you can make healthy choices at your meals and snacks.

At first, this may be somewhat daunting—calculating and precisely measuring every food you eat never sounds like a lot of fun. But like so many other things about starting on a pump, it will become routine and you will eventually remember the carb content of the foods you eat most often, as well as what constitutes a serving size. The benefits of your diligence in the beginning will definitely pay off in the long run.

THE FOOD LABEL: THE OLD AND THE NEW

Reading a food label is a key skill for managing blood glucose levels and carb counting successfully. There are four things that you must always look at when you read a nutrition or food label. These are:

- serving size
- total fat
- total carbohydrates
- dietary fiber

In the new food label, there is an additional line indicating added sugars.

Nutrition Facts

Serving Size 2/3 cup (55g)
Servings Per Container About 8

Amount Per Serving

Calories 230   Calories from Fat 72

	% Daily Value*
Total Fat 8g	**12%**
Saturated Fat 1g	**5%**
Trans Fat 0g	
Cholesterol 0mg	**0%**
Sodium 160mg	**7%**
Total Carbohydrate 37g	**12%**
Dietary Fiber 4g	**16%**
Sugars 1g	
Protein 3g	
Vitamin A	10%
Vitamin C	8%
Calcium	20%
Iron	45%

*Percent Daily Values are based on a 2,000 calorie diet.
Your Daily Values may be higher or lower depending on
your calorie needs.

	Calories:	2,000	2,500
Total Fat	Less than	65g	80g
Sat Fat	Less than	20g	25g
Cholesterol	Less than	300mg	300mg
Sodium	Less than	2,400mg	2,400mg
Potassium		3,500mg	3,500mg
Total Carbohydrate		300g	375g
Dietary Fiber		25g	30g

Nutrition Facts

8 servings per container

Serving size   **2/3 cup (55g)**

Amount per serving

Calories   **230**

	% Daily Value*
Total Fat 8g	**10%**
Saturated Fat 1g	**5%**
Trans Fat 0g	
Cholesterol 0mg	**0%**
Sodium 160mg	**7%**
Total Carbohydrate 37g	**13%**
Dietary Fiber 4g	**14%**
Total Sugars 12g	
Includes 10g Added Sugars	**20%**
Protein 3g	
Vitamin D 2mcg	10%
Calcium 260mcg	20%
Iron 8mg	45%
Potassium 235mg	6%

*The % Daily Value (DV) tells you how much a nutrient in a
serving of food contributes to a daily diet. 2,000 calories
a day is used for general nutrition advice.

OLD   **NEW**

Let's look at food labels together. The examples we use are for ice cream. The best idea is to start at the top of the food label.

Serving Size

What is the serving size here? This label shows the serving size for 2/3 cup of ice cream. Knowing this is essential because all of the rest of the nutrient content is based on a single serving of the food. The next time you grab a bag of chips, look closely at how many servings are in the bag. The label will tell you right under the serving size. For bagels, there might be six bagels in a bag. Each bagel is one serving. Serving sizes often give the amount in weight and/or volume. Some labels will indicate a measurement, such as 1/2 cup, as well as a weight in ounces (oz) or grams. Liquid serving sizes are generally in fluid ounces (oz), cups, or milliliters (mL). In this case, the weight of the ice cream serving is 55 grams. These weight grams are different from the grams of carbohydrate in the serving, so be careful not to mix them up! *If a label indicated that the serving size is a half bagel, then you'd have to double all of the nutrients in the food label if you eat the whole bagel.*

Total Fat

The next thing to look at is total fat. This ice cream serving has 8 grams of fat. If you look at the line right above the total fat line, you will see the percent of the daily value.

More About Fats

The 2017 American Diabetes Association (ADA) Standards of Care recommend that the type of fats you consume is as important as the amount of fat you eat as your percentage of total calories. It is recommended that you eat about 20–35% of your total calories as mainly monounsaturated fats (plant-based fats like olive oil and sesame oil) and little saturated fats (animal fats and fats found in butter and cheese). The ADA acknowledges that a Mediterranean-style diet may be an effective way to lower your risk of cardiovascular disease, if it replaces a diet with low fat and high carbohydrate content. The Mediterranean diet is higher in monounsaturated fats and lower in total carbohydrates.

Many people now also follow a higher–monounsaturated fat, lower-carbohydrate diet. There is evidence that individuals do experience improved glycemic control by significantly lowering their carbohydrate intake and limiting their carbohydrates to mostly non-starchy vegetables (e.g., greens, cucumbers, broccoli, cauliflower, Brussels sprouts, and lettuce). With this lower-carb diet, calories from carbs are replaced with those from fat. The body prefers carbohydrates for energy, but it can also use fat for energy. You do not want a nutrition plan that is both high in fat and high in carbohydrates, since this can lead to weight gain and insulin resistance. The

ANOTHER THING ABOUT FAT

Fat delays the emptying of your stomach. Therefore, it takes longer for food to digest and have an effect on your glucose level. You might want to consider using a dual-wave or square-wave bolus if you eat high-fat foods (foods or meals with about 30% or more calories from fat).

The higher the fat content of a meal, the longer the duration of the square wave of the meal bolus. For example, for pizza, you might want to take 50% of the insulin dosage immediately and 50% as the square wave over 4 hours. For fried food, take 50% immediately and 50% over 2 hours. For ice cream, take 70% immediately and 30% over 2 hours. The dosage is determined by the total carbohydrate content of the meal, and then if the 2-hour glucose level is low, put more insulin in the square wave next time. If the 2-hour glucose is high, give more insulin immediately next time.

response to a high-fat diet with regard to insulin dosage is variable; some individuals require less insulin and others require more.

Some people start a very-low-carb or ketogenic diet to lose weight. This tactic works for some people, but the ADA does not recognize any one macronutrient exclusion as superior for weight loss. Particularly if you have type 1 diabetes, the long-term effect of elevating your ketone levels by restricting dietary carbohydrate and increasing fat intake is not known. What is most important for weight loss is the total amount of calories eaten compared to energy expended.

Total Carbohydrate

Total carbohydrate gives you the total amount of carbohydrate, including sugar and fiber, in the food. For this ice cream, total carbohydrate is 37 grams. If you were using a CR of 8 (1 unit for every 8 grams of carbohydrate), the total amount of insulin needed to cover this ice cream serving would be 4.62 units (37 grams of carbohydrate ÷ 8 CR = 4.60 units of insulin and rounded up or down to either 4.60 or 4.65 units). If you were still on MDI, you wouldn't be able to take 4.60 units of insulin. You would have to round down to 4 units or up to 5 units (unless you had half-unit syringes, in which case you could take 4.5 units). With an insulin pump, you can administer these small increments, as low as 0.025 units. For some people, these small increments are necessary to fine-tune insulin delivery.

When looking at the total carbohydrate content, keep in mind the serving size! If, for example, you eat only half a bagel, then you will need to take only half the amount of insulin.

Dietary Fiber

Next look at the dietary fiber. This ice cream has 4 grams of fiber. It is important to have fiber in your diet, and foods high in fiber are usually healthy choices. Fruits and vegetables are naturally high in fiber. Whole grains contain higher amounts of fiber than processed grains. Because fiber is not digested completely in your gastrointestinal tract, fiber has little effect on your glucose levels. If you eat a food with more than 5 grams of fiber, you can subtract the grams of fiber from the total grams of carbohydrate for the carb number you will use with your CR. For example, if a bagel had 7 grams of fiber, you would subtract 7 grams from 50 grams to get 43 grams, and 43 grams would be the total number of carbs you would use in the CR. With a CR of 15, you would take 2.85 units of insulin for the bagel with 7 grams of fiber. In general, high-fiber foods don't elevate your blood glucose as much as foods without fiber. In this example, you do not need to subtract the fiber from your carb count.

Finally, in the new food label, it tells you how much of the carbohydrate is from added sugars. The less the added sugar, the better.

Protein

You should also check the amount of protein in the food you are choosing. Protein is an essential nutrient, but many people eat too much of it. Try to get 20–25% of your daily calories from protein. If you have kidney disease, you should aim for the lower end of that range. Note that there is not enough scientific evidence to suggest that a high-protein (and high-fat), low-carbohydrate diet is helpful in managing diabetes. However, there are increasing numbers of

IF YOU CAN'T FIND A FOOD LABEL

Although the food label is a useful thing to have so that you can more effectively manage your diabetes, not every food has one. When was the last time you saw a food label on fresh fruit, a hamburger, or a restaurant meal? There are many foods that you will encounter every day that will not have a label, but there are other ways to get the nutrition facts you need to help determine your insulin requirements. Most chain and fast-food restaurants have their nutrition facts online and in pamphlets at the restaurant. If you are lucky, those details will be right there on the menu. Sometimes this information is hidden away, but if you ask for it, you can see it. There are many books that have the nutrition facts for a variety of restaurants. Such books are generally small or pocket-size and portable. Bring them with you when you are out and about. There are also many apps for phones that have total nutrition content for a wide variety of foods, including menus from restaurants. These display calories, fat, protein, carbs, and fiber values and will change based on the serving size you choose.

people with type 1 diabetes who are restricting their carbohydrate intake and eating more protein (and fat). For those who eat more grams of protein than grams of carbohydrate, they can consider counting the grams of protein, divide the grams by 50%, and then take insulin per their CR for half of the protein grams with a square wave over a 6-hour time period.

A VALUABLE RESOURCE

In addition to the nearly countless online resources for nutrition information, you can also carry this information with you at all times. Pick up a copy of *The Diabetes Carbohydrate & Fat Gram Guide*, 5th edition, by Lea Ann Holzmeister, published by the American Diabetes Association, or *Eat Out, Eat Well—The Guide to Eating Healthy at Any Restaurant*, 4th edition, by Hope S. Warshaw, also published by the American Diabetes Association.

CONDIMENTS COUNT!

Don't forget to count the carbs in any toppings you use. Ketchup, jelly, hot sauces, and BBQ sauce often have significant numbers of carbs per serving. If you feel like your CR is correct and you counted all the carbs in the foods, but your postmeal glucose was higher than expected, maybe you forgot to count the carbs in the condiments, toppings, and sauces.

IMPORTANCE OF ACCURATE MEASUREMENTS

In addition to knowing the number of carbohydrates in each serving of the foods you eat, taking accurate measurements of how much you actually eat is an important part of counting carbs. If the amount you actually eat does not equal what you thought you ate, then your bolus will be incorrect. Measuring is important, but it can definitely be difficult. Here are some tips that will help you get started with measuring accurately:

- Some items need to be measured by weight or by volume. A food scale will be best for weighing things like bread or meat. A scale can also be used for fruits and pasta—the serving size for pasta is usually 2 oz, but this is almost always 2 oz before it is cooked. Be sure to check your pasta label to determine if the information is for dry or for cooked pasta. Measuring cups can be good for grains and cereals, graduated cups are good for liquids (bend down, so that you are at eye level with the measurements), and teaspoons and tablespoons are good for jams, honey, butter, and peanut butter.

- Always level off what's in your measuring utensil with a knife.

- Check to see if the food label or the book indicates raw versus cooked, because this distinction can change the composition of the food's nutrition content. This is often the case for pasta and grains (rice, quinoa, popcorn).

- Watch your portion sizes as you grow more confident in your ability to estimate. If your glucose numbers are rising, go back to carefully measuring your foods. Often, as time passes, we lose track of what a true serving looks like. If this happens to you, it's time to go back and recalibrate your visual measuring skills.

- Start to notice what different foods look like on your plate. This step will be helpful when you go out to eat and don't have a measuring cup or scale handy. There are some good ways to estimate size, but it is still important to keep measuring every so often to keep your estimates accurate.

- There are some easy ways to estimate what you're eating by comparing them to familiar objects. Using this system, 3 oz of meat is about the size of a deck of playing cards. A 1/2 cup of pasta, rice, or grains is about the size of your palm, whereas 1 cup is the size of your fist. A medium potato is the size of a computer mouse. With fruits, a "small" piece would be about the size of a tennis ball and 1/2 cup is about the size of a baseball. A tablespoon of peanut butter and other similar foods is about equal to the size of your thumb. A teaspoon is about the size of the tip of your thumb. A small cup of coffee is about 8 oz or 1 cup of liquid. An ounce of cheese is about the size of three dice.

Sometimes foods come with a volume and a weight measurement. If you find that your carb counting works sometimes but not others, try measuring your food by weight rather than volume. You might be surprised at how much more food is in the volume measurement versus that measurement by weight. For things like maple syrup, this difference could mean a few carbs!

GLYCEMIC INDEX

The glycemic index is a meal-planning tool based on how quickly the carbohydrates in a food will affect blood glucose levels. While once a preferred way to assess carbohydrate quality, it is not used much now. Foods are listed on a scale of 1–100, with 100 being a food that affects your blood glucose the fastest. Pure glucose is the fastest carbohydrate in terms of reaching the blood and has a glycemic index of 100. All other foods are compared to this. Low-glycemic foods are generally considered 55 and under, whereas high-glycemic foods are above 75. Be aware, however, that the glycemic index of a food does not affect the total amount of insulin you take. It is not a carbohydrate count. A slice of sourdough bread has a glycemic index of 52, but four slices have four times the amount of carbohydrate as one slice. Therefore, you will need to take four times more insulin, even though the glycemic index remained 52.

Timing of Insulin Delivery

The carbohydrate quality, simple versus complex carbs, helps you plan the timing of insulin delivery. It is already a good idea to take your insulin 15–30 minutes before you eat a meal, but taking your insulin early for a meal that is going to have a lot of simple carbs is particularly effective for managing blood glucose levels. However, foods composed of complex carbs, and particularly when mixed with foods with a high fat content, may take longer to reach your bloodstream and might need insulin administered over a longer period of time. A square-wave or dual-wave bolus would be a good option here. Foods like pasta are often treated with a dual-wave bolus because an initial burst of insulin is needed to cover the first glucose spike as the food is first digested. But because the carbs will take longer to reach the bloodstream, insulin delivery will also have to be drawn out, making the dual-wave bolus the ideal solution.

Things that affect timing of glucose absorption include fat; any coating on the food, such as in waxy beans and legumes; ripeness (the sugar content in many fruits and vegetables increases with age); type of starch; fiber content; acidity (it slows digestion); processing; cooking methods; and your before-meal glucose level. Processed grains have had the bran and germ removed, which reduces the content of natural nutrients like fiber, resulting in more rapid absorption. With cooking, the longer you cook a food, the faster it reaches the bloodstream. This happens because the cooking process starts to break down the carbohydrate in the food, making it easier for the body to absorb it.

ALCOHOL

Alcohol and mixers can affect glucose levels both at the time you drink them and 16–24 hours later. Adults who drink need to know that alcohol can drop glucose levels several hours after ingestion because of the effect alcohol has on the liver and other hormones in the body. Normally, the liver is putting out small amounts of glucose (which is why you need a basal rate), but when the liver is processing alcohol, it stops producing glucose or drops the amount. This process can lead to a hypoglycemic episode if basal rates are not adjusted. In a person without diabetes, the pancreas will drop insulin levels to account for the drop in glucose, but a person with diabetes needs to be conscious of this and either prepare a new basal rate, set a temporary basal rate, or eat food and carbs to decrease the chance of a low glucose level (or maybe a combination of all of these). If you are drinking in the evening, you are at greater risk for nighttime low glucose levels.

> One type of alcohol may cause regular and predictable low glucose levels, while another may not cause hypoglycemia. The amount of alcohol can also affect glucose levels.

Mixers and certain types of alcohol also contain a fair number of carbs. Beer, margaritas, hard cider, and soda mixers (unless diet) will cause your glucose to spike at the time you drink it. However, you may still have a drop in glucose levels later. Many people find

It is also a good idea to eat foods with protein or fat along with carbs before or when drinking. These foods will help keep glucose levels in safe ranges. Remember to drink water as well!

that if they take a normal amount of bolus for the carbs in alcohol, their glucose levels drop later; therefore, they decrease their initial bolus amount or don't take a bolus. Straight/hard alcohol (e.g., bourbon, gin, rum, or tequila) and dry or red wines have few carbs and often do not require a bolus. Darker beers, hard ciders, sweet wine, and mixed drinks may need a bolus.

Some alcohols may affect your blood glucose values differently. One type of alcohol may cause regular and predictable low glucose levels, while another may not cause hypoglycemia. The amount of alcohol can also affect glucose levels. (The ADA recommends that adult males do not drink more than two drinks in a day and adult women no more than one drink.) If consuming a moderate amount of alcohol, it is wise to be cautious and use a temporary basal that is a reduced rate (20% reduction; 80% of your normal amount) overnight before going to bed, or make sure you eat a snack. If you are active while you drink (e.g., dancing), a temporary basal rate of approximately 50% overnight might be recommended. Set a reminder to wake up after a few hours and check your glucose. If you have a CGM, make sure your alerts are audible.

Sometimes the effect of alcohol mimics hypoglycemia, and it is easy to mistake or miss a low blood glucose level. If you are out drinking, check glucose levels often and tell someone that you have diabetes. It is suggested that someone in your group refrain from

Avoid drinking after a day with vigorous exercise. High activity levels increase the chance of hypoglycemia.

drinking and understand your risk of hypoglycemia. Otherwise, if you have a hypoglycemic episode and require help, others may not take the situation seriously.

Hypoglycemia caused by alcohol can be harder to treat, or it may require more glucose to adequately bring up your glucose levels. Place a source of glucose within reach before you fall asleep so that you have access to it if you wake up with a low glucose reaction.

As always, if you choose to drink alcohol, please do so wisely and safely.

CHAPTER REVIEW

➡ Carbohydrate counting is the preferred meal-planning tool for someone using an insulin pump. Compared with other methods, counting carbs is easier and more precise, once you determine your CR.

➡ Carbohydrates come in three forms: starches, sugars, and fiber. A gram of starch or sugar is counted as a gram of carbohydrate. Fiber is counted differently. Fiber is not completely digested or converted to glucose. If there is a large portion of fiber in your meal (5 or more grams), then you can subtract the number of grams of fiber from the total carbohydrate count.

➡ There are four key elements to look at when you read a food label. These are serving size, total fat, total carbohydrates, and dietary fiber.

➡ If you do not know how much you eat or drink, you will not be able to accurately calculate how much insulin you need to take. Measuring is important! But measuring is also not always easy because there is not one way that works to measure every food you eat. With practice, you will become familiar with portion sizes.

➡ Alcohol can cause hypoglycemia. If you choose to drink, makes sure to eat a meal with carbohydrates before drinking, modify your basal rates or eat a snack before bed, and wake up in the night to check glucose levels. Please drink responsibly.

IN THIS CHAPTER

CHAPTER 7

UNDERSTANDING THE IMPACT OF PHYSICAL ACTIVITY

Hopefully, you are physically active and have regular exercise as a part of your daily routine. Exercise not only helps your metabolism, but also helps you maintain a healthy weight and is good for your heart, your muscles, your bones, and your mood, whether or not you have diabetes. It doesn't matter if you are an athlete or someone who rarely gets off the couch; you can use your insulin pump to keep your glucose levels under control with exercise—particularly if your activity varies in intensity and duration from one day to the next. A continuous glucose monitor (CGM) may help you understand the glucose effects of your usual exercise routines; to spot impending high or low glucose levels before, during, and after exercise; and to manage unexpected bouts of activity more effectively. Understanding how to manage planned and unplanned physical activity is important for a successful journey with diabetes and with insulin pump therapy.

To be active doesn't mean you have to run marathons or put in

GET MOVIN'!

It is recommended that adults should engage in 150 minutes of moderate-to-vigorous exercise spread over at least 3 days/week, with no more than 2 consecutive days without activity. For children, it is recommended to have 60 minutes per day of moderate-to-vigorous exercise. So get out and get movin' for your health!

long hours at the gym. You can take a walk at lunch or after school. You can dance, bike to the store, work in your garden, wash your car, and routinely take the stairs instead of the elevator. Even standing for parts of the day instead of sitting will help. Do your best to move your body as much as possible, and you and your diabetes will reap the benefits.

JUST STARTING OUT

When you first get your pump and you're trying to determine how to set your bolus and basal rates, you actually don't want to do excessive exercise, even if you are someone who exercises routinely. It is easier to determine your pump settings when you are sedentary (i.e., not very physically active). Once you establish your ratios and feel comfortable with your pump, you can start being more active again.

Start slowly and exercise for a shorter period of time than usual. For example, if you routinely exercise for 45–60 minutes several times a week, start out at 20–30 minutes. Once you figure out how to manage these shorter periods of activity, you can increase your exercise by 15–20 minutes, until you get to your typical exercise duration. You can do the same with intensity. Start with a lower intensity until you get the hang of how to manage your glucose and insulin levels during exercise. After that, you can move up the intensity ladder. In the end, you will succeed in being active and having optimal glucose control.

Exercise Physiology

Hypoglycemia is a risk of exercise. The more you exercise, the more sensitive to insulin you will become. Being more sensitive to insulin means you might need to take less insulin overall. Exercise helps increase the number of insulin receptors on cells. When insulin attaches to these receptors, glucose can pass from the blood into the cell. This reduces the amount of glucose in the blood, which can lead to hypoglycemia.

Your muscles use carbohydrate and fat. Once food is absorbed and the resulting glucose is used up, your body relies on its own

WHEN STARTING TO EXERCISE, ALWAYS THINK ABOUT . . .

- The type, intensity, and duration of your activity
- Your starting glucose level
- Your starting basal rate
- When you took your last bolus (to know how much active insulin is present)
- The last time you had food
- The time of day
- Where your infusion set is placed on your body
- Your hydration level

stores. At the beginning of exercise, the muscles use their own glucose stores (glucose is stored as glycogen in muscle tissue). Then, glucose is released from the liver. At this point, people who do not have diabetes have a sharp drop in their insulin levels and a rise in their epinephrine (or adrenaline) levels. This process triggers fat stores to release fatty acids, another fuel source. If exercise continues, muscles use more and more fatty acids for fuel; by 40 minutes or so, fatty acids account for 35% of the fuel used by muscles, and by 4 hours, they account for 70%.

In someone with diabetes, if insulin levels do not decrease, glucose and fatty acids are not released from the body's stores. Hypoglycemia will be a big risk. Even after exercise, muscles continue to use up glucose, glycogen stores are not replenished, and muscles are more sensitive to insulin, so hypoglycemia is still a risk.

In addition, you need to follow your glucose levels, determine your carbohydrate intake, and adjust your insulin levels while you are active and after you are done. If your infusion set is placed in your leg or arm and you do not have a lot of tissue there, your cannula may be closer to your muscles, resulting in your insulin being absorbed faster than if it were in a more fatty location (like your abdomen). You may notice that you are more prone to hypoglycemia during exercise if your set is in a muscular area.

GLUCOSE LEVELS BEFORE, DURING, AND AFTER EXERCISE

Before you exercise, you need to check your glucose level.

Starting with Low Glucose

If your glucose level is low (<70 mg/dL), then you need to correct it by ingesting carbohydrate before you begin exercising. You will need 15–30 grams of carbohydrate. Wait 15 minutes, and then check your glucose level again. You might not want to start exercising until your glucose is >100 mg/dL. Consider decreasing your basal insulin before or during exercise. It is important to check your glucose levels at least every 30–60 minutes. If there is a downward trend, you will need to ingest some carbohydrate to avoid hypoglycemia; if you catch it soon enough, suspending insulin may also help. A CGM can help during exercise and can determine if you need additional glucose or whether suspending or reducing basal rates before exercise is sufficient to avoid hypoglycemia. The trend arrows on a CGM allow you to see if glucose levels are dropping and at what rate. In addition, if your glucose levels are trending upward, you may choose not to suspend or decrease your basal insulin before exercise.

Quick-acting or simple carbohydrates are the best for elevating your glucose level. Glucose tabs, glucose gels, icing, juice, or a sports drink (make sure it contains sugar, not a diet one) are all rapidly absorbed and good choices for quick boosts during exercise. They are also better options than solid foods that contain carbohydrate, such as snack bars, fruit, breads, crackers, or protein, because glucose raises blood glucose faster. Solid foods are better for sustaining glucose levels over long periods of exercise, or once you have already treated a low glucose level with fast-acting carbs and are in the safe-to-exercise zone again.

Starting in Target

If your glucose level is in the target range before you begin your activity, then you should follow your usual exercise routine in terms of duration and intensity. The trend of glucose levels immediately

REMEMBER! IT IS *NOT* SAFE TO EXERCISE WITH KETONES!

before exercise may indicate how the glucose levels will respond during exercise. For instance, if glucose levels are decreasing immediately before exercise, they will probably continue to decrease during exercise, indicating that adjustment of basal rates or extra glucose ingestion may be indicated.

Starting with High Glucose

If your glucose is >250 mg/dL, then you need to check for ketones before starting exercise. You should not exercise when you have ketones because of the risk of diabetic ketoacidosis (DKA). A high glucose level indicates a lack of insulin or insulin effect, and activity can cause your liver to release stored glucose and cause your blood glucose to climb even higher. Physical activity can lead your body to begin burning fat, which leads to ketone formation. If your glucose is between 250 and 300 mg/dL, you don't have ketones, and you decide to continue with your activity, then be very cautious. Take a correction bolus first (it should probably be smaller than the actual bolus calculated by your pump; this is covered later in this chapter), and check your glucose every 30–60 minutes or watch your CGM to make sure your level is improving and not dropping too quickly.

Low Glucose Levels During and After Exercise

You should plan on checking glucose levels every 30–60 minutes while you exercise. Your exercise intensity and duration and your starting glucose level will give you an idea of how frequently you will need to check. If your glucose level is decreasing, you can decrease or stop your basal insulin by using the temporary basal rate or suspend feature on your pump. You can also ingest carbohydrate or do both: change your insulin dose and take carbs.

You need to check your glucose level after you are finished with activity and more frequently through the rest of the day and night; alternatively, a CGM will show you if you begin to trend down. You can anticipate that glucose levels might be low after exercise (even hours later). You can help prevent or treat lows by using temporary basal rates, temporarily suspending basal insulin (if you continue to get low), or consuming extra carbohydrate without covering it with a bolus. If you do give a bolus, decrease the insulin dose so that your carb intake effectively treats your hypoglycemia and it does not completely cover all of the carbohydrates.

Hyperglycemia After Exercise

You might find that your glucose level is high during or after exercise, perhaps much higher than when you started. Elevated glucose at these times is due to the release of epinephrine (also called adrenaline) and other hormones that help release stored glucose. Intense workouts, such as sprints or weight training, can cause a surge of adrenaline and these other hormones. You should usually avoid taking a correction dose of insulin during your workout, because, as exercise continues, high blood glucose levels often drop and can actually turn into low blood glucose levels. However, if you have decreased your basal rate, you might want to return to your usual level if hyperglycemia persists for over 1 hour. If your glucose is very high, you might want to consider taking a small correction dosage.

Your activity may not need a decrease in insulin, but rather an increase to correct glucose levels, especially if your sport activity involves an increase in adrenaline. If your glucose levels increase during your activity but a regular correction bolus causes hypoglycemia, try a partial correction as a square-wave bolus over 30–60 minutes, for the duration of the last half of your session.

After you have completed your workout, if your blood glucose levels are still high and stay that way for over 1–2 hours, you should consider taking a correction bolus, but reduce it by 50%. If you continue to have hyperglycemia, you might consider a 75–100% correction bolus after another 2–3 hours.

ADJUST YOUR INSULIN

You usually need to reduce your basal rate when you exercise. Again, depending on the length and the intensity, you might reduce your basal insulin before, during, and after exercise or even suspend basal insulin altogether. Depending on the intensity and duration of the physical activity, you might also need to reduce the boluses you give for your meal before exercise and for the extra carbohydrate you eat before, during, and after exercise. Some of those carbs may be taken without administering insulin at all.

The most common way to help prevent hypoglycemia is to reduce the amount of insulin you receive in both your basal rates and your boluses (for both food and correction). Even if you disconnect your pump for contact sports or water activities, you must have some amount of active insulin. So how do you do this? Some of it is trial and error, but there are some overall principles of how to start.

Exercise and Basal Rates

Here are some tips on getting started with adjusting your basal insulin levels for exercise. Remember, your basal rate will need to be adjusted depending on the duration and intensity of the physical activity.

- **Mild activity.** You might need a reduction like 5–25% (75–95% of your regular rate) if you are doing mild exercise, such as gardening, vacuuming, or washing the car. If you are normally fairly active, you may not need a reduction for this type of activity.

- **Moderate activity.** For any activity that makes you sweat after about 10 minutes or makes you breathe harder, you may need a 25–50% reduction in basal rates (50–75% of your regular rate).

- **High-intensity activity.** If you plan on high-intensity exercise, a 50–100% reduction or complete disconnection from the pump may be needed. Try different basal reductions for different durations. Check your glucose often.

- **Downward trends.** If your glucose tends to head downward during any exercise, then you should consider another 25–50% reduction in your basal rate while exercising.

- **Zero basal rate.** If you want to eliminate basal insulin delivery altogether, you can either disconnect your pump or keep it on with a temporary basal rate of 0% for the duration of the exercise. By using a basal rate and keeping your pump connected, there is no chance that you will forget to reconnect when you are done exercising. Don't forget that if your activity lasts longer than 1 hour, you'll need to check your glucose and determine whether you need to take a dose of insulin to replace your lost basal rate, once your exercise is complete. If you do suspend or disconnect your pump, it is not recommended to do that for more than 2 hours without restarting insulin delivery.

- **Amount of time.** The amount of time you plan on exercising might also affect your basal rate reduction. If you plan on doing a very short exercise session, less than 15–30 minutes, you might not need to reduce basal rates. However, for more moderate periods of time, you might want to consider a significant reduction or disconnection of the pump. If you plan on doing long, strenuous, or continuous exercise (such as running or jogging, all-day hikes, or all-day sport competitions), then a very small basal rate, such as a 20% basal (80% reduction), might be a good idea to avoid forming ketones. With this type of long-term activity and continued insulin delivery, it is important to eat snacks along the way to keep ingesting carbohydrates to avoid hypoglycemia. Drinking sports drinks with carbohydrates as well as water throughout will help you stay hydrated and give you glucose.

- **Your exercise pattern.** If you are someone who exercises frequently and/or for long periods of time, you may not need as drastic a decrease in your basal rates, particularly for mild exercise. Your body may already be accustomed to this type of exercise and significant reductions might cause hyperglycemia.

- **Start basal reduction before exercise.** Depending on the type, intensity, and duration of your exercise, you might want to start reducing basal insulin rates 30–60 minutes before you begin activity. This step will enable you to start exercising with a reduced level of insulin in your bloodstream, which helps prevent hypo-glycemia.

• **Delayed hypoglycemia and basal reduction.** Exercise may cause delayed hypoglycemia. This is especially a concern if you exercise in the afternoon, which might increase your risk of hypoglycemia during the night. Using temporary basal rates through the night can help reduce the risk of hypoglycemia. For example, you might consider a basal rate reduction of about 20% for the hours of 10:00 P.M. to 6:00 A.M. (this means you will be given 80% of your usual basal rate). Once this temporary rate is in place, wake up once or twice during the night and check your glucose levels to see if the reduction is working, or use a CGM.

  Delayed hypoglycemia is also common after long, strenuous workouts, like hiking, marathons, or anything that lasts 2 or more hours. If you are doing a long stretch of exercise, you might also consider decreasing your basal rates as soon as you stop being active. A 20% reduction in basal rates for 2–3 hours after you finish might also reduce the risk of hypoglycemia.

• **Post-exercise hyperglycemia.** Post-exercise hyperglycemia can happen if you sprint or do exercises that increase your levels of stress hormones. Other common activities that can cause post-exercise hyperglycemia include competitions (due to elevation of adrenaline) and weightlifting. For these, you might find doing a small bolus of 0.5–1.0 units halfway through the workout can help keep glucose levels from rising. If you are running a race and sprint the last part, you may notice a sharp increase in glucose levels. Small boluses can be given as you start the sprint, or, once you cross the finish line, you can increase your basal insulin rate. Trying these different options will give you a good idea about what works best for reducing your post-exercise high glucose levels.

• **Separate basal pattern.** If you are part of a sports team or do the same type of exercise routinely every day, a new basal pattern is probably a good idea. Switching to this "exercise" pattern for the days you plan on being active gives you consistency, convenience, and freedom.

KNOW YOUR INTENSITY LEVEL

➡ **Low:** You can talk and sing. You don't sweat, and you have no trouble breathing.

➡ **Moderate:** Your breathing is harder, and you can no longer sing, although you can talk.

➡ **High:** No singing or talking. You begin to sweat very soon after starting the activity.

Correction Doses and Exercise

Depending on what your glucose level is before you begin activity, and what you plan on doing and for how long, you will need to adjust how much insulin you give to correct a glucose level above your target range. You might consider a 50–100% reduction (a 100% reduction means no insulin at all). In general, for mild exercise that doesn't last very long (e.g., mowing the lawn or a leisurely walk around a park), if your starting glucose is above 180 mg/dL, then you might not need a reduction, or you might only need a small reduction (about 25%). If you plan on doing more moderate exercise or for longer periods of time, and your glucose is 100–180 mg/dL, a 50–75% reduction is a good idea. The table below shows some guidelines for how to correct a glucose level that is above target.

Change a correction bolus if it is taken 60–90 minutes before you start to exercise.

How to Change a Correction Bolus Before Exercise

Exercise Duration (in minutes)	Intensity	Blood glucose level (mg/dL)	Possible decrease in bolus (% decrease)
<30	Mild	≥180*	50
		100–180	50–75
30–60	Moderate	≥180*	50–75
		100–180	75–100
≥60	Intense	≥180*	50–85
		100–180	85–100

*If your blood glucose level is above 250 mg/dL and you have ketones, DO NOT EXERCISE.

Food Boluses

You often need to ingest carbohydrate before you exercise, while you are exercising (if it is of long duration), and after you are done. You decide what amount, frequency, and kind of carbohydrate to eat depending on the length and intensity of the exercise and how you feel after eating different foods, such as snack bars and drinks. Some of this you will have to learn through trial and error.

Reducing basal and bolus amounts may not be enough to prevent hypoglycemia during exercise. Many people must also eat before or during activity or both to keep their blood glucose up, so they start with a 50% reduction in food boluses.

Generally, people start with about 15 grams of carbohydrate from a liquid source, such as sports drinks, juice, or even milk (which has protein, too), before starting their activity, although make sure you drink something that won't upset your stomach. These liquid carbs can last for about 30 minutes of moderate exercise and hit the bloodstream faster than carbohydrates from solid food and protein. Solid foods and foods that contain protein are absorbed more slowly and can help keep glucose levels elevated longer. If you are planning on doing a short amount of exercise, such as 30 minutes or less, and you have a blood glucose level within target (around 120 mg/dL), then you may not need extra carbohydrates. If you do, you can drink 15 grams of carbohydrate, and you may not need to take any extra insulin. If you plan on doing more sustained exercise, such as an hour or more, then you may need to eat solid carbohydrates, too. This might include a half sandwich (or whole sandwich, depending on what the activity is) with protein, such as meat or cheese. If you cannot exercise with a full stomach, eat your meal about 30–45 minutes before exercising so you have time to digest, and then reduce your bolus per the planned duration and intensity of your activity.

When eating before exercise, it might be necessary to reduce your bolus even up to 60–90 minutes before your activity depending on its intensity. A strenuous walk may be enough to cause a low sugar when there is insulin-on-board (IOB) from a meal 1–1.5 hours earlier. Adjusting food boluses before exercise is also related to how and when insulin peaks in the body. Eating 90 minutes to 2 hours before your exercise may not need a reduction because the insulin has already peaked and is starting to be reduced. However, if you still have IOB, then you still have extra insulin that may cause a low glucose reaction. Reducing boluses this far out may only need about a 20% reduction. This step will effectively decrease the IOB before exercise. The closer you get to your exercise time, the more you should decrease your bolus amount (this includes bolus insulin for both food and correction). A bolus within 30–45 minutes of exercise hasn't hit the peak efficiency, and there will be much more IOB, meaning there is a much higher likelihood of hypoglycemia. Remember, activity increases muscle uptake of glucose. Any extra insulin around will allow more glucose to be used than when you are not exercising. A good place to start is to decrease your bolus starting 90 minutes before exercise. At 90 minutes, take 75% of your bolus (or decrease it by 25%); at 60 minutes, take 50% of your bolus (or decrease it by 50%); and at 30 minutes, reduce it to 25% (or decrease it by 75%). However, for many people, a reduction greater than 50% is too much. If you are going to reduce your bolus amount before exercise, then check your glucose value before you start exercising.

Use your CGM to help you understand when your insulin peaks and how fast your blood glucose drops if you have IOB during exercise. If you tend to do the same activity, make sure to upload your CGM and look at the way your glucose levels respond to your bolus or basal changes.

Treating Lows During and After Exercise

Even if you have reduced your basal rates and correction boluses and have eaten, hypoglycemia still happens. Treating it may need to be a little more vigorous than the usual 15 grams of carbohydrate that you normally take for an everyday low. Thirty grams of carbohydrate may need to be eaten first and 15 grams more if you plan on doing more intense exercise after you recover. *It is important that you do not continue to exercise if your blood glucose levels have not increased.* After eating, wait 15 minutes and then test again. If you still have not seen a rise in your blood glucose, eat 15 grams of carbohydrate and wait another 15 minutes. Be sure to always have snacks and quick-acting carbs handy (e.g., glucose tabs or juice) when you exercise!

A FEW FINAL THOUGHTS

- Safety is essential when it comes to exercise. Be prepared for hypoglycemia and hyperglycemia. Tell people around you what to do and how to help you in case of an emergency. If you are part of a sports team, inform your coach or some close teammates about what to do if you are unable to treat yourself. Let them know where your supplies are and how to administer them.

- Drink plenty of water! Dehydration can increase the chance of ketones and make it harder to get rid of them if they develop. A healthy body is a hydrated body. You may need to drink carbohydrates during your workout to keep your glucose in the target range.

- If you are exercising outside on a hot day, bring a cooler to put your pump and supplies in so that they don't overheat in the sun. If you go on a long bike ride or hike, position your pump on the side of your body that might be shaded. If insulin gets too hot, it can lose its effectiveness. Intense heat may also damage your pump! If this happens and you don't have a backup insulin source, you are likely to develop high blood glucose levels and can potentially develop ketones. Always have a plan for your activity that includes backup insulin and plenty of glucose/snacks.

- Once you start exercising and continue to do it regularly, and especially if you lose weight, you will most likely need less insulin for your daily life. If you start to notice more frequent hypoglycemia on days you are not exercising, you may need to reduce your basal rates, carbohydrate ratio, or insulin sensitivity factor to accommodate for being more insulin sensitive. This is a good thing! Increasing insulin sensitivity is an outcome of increased physical activity. Reach out to your diabetes health care team if you feel like you need many changes at once.

CHAPTER REVIEW

➡ Hypoglycemia is a risk of exercise. The more you exercise, the more sensitive to insulin you will become. Being more sensitive to insulin means you might need to take less insulin overall. And not just while you are exercising, but hours later and in the night.

➡ When you start to exercise, you always need to think about the following: the type, intensity, and duration of your activity; your starting glucose; your starting basal rate; when you took your last bolus (so you know how much active insulin is in your body); the last time you ate or had carbs; the time of day; where your infusion set is placed on your body; and your hydration level. Do not exercise if you have ketones.

➡ Check your glucose level every 30–60 minutes while you exercise. The more intense the exercise is, the longer its duration, and the lower your starting glucose, the more often you need to check. Treat low glucose levels. You need to measure your glucose level after you are done being active and more frequently through the rest of the day and night. You can anticipate that glucose levels might be low even hours after exercise. Be aware that you might find your glucose level is high during or after exercise, possibly much higher than when you started. Elevated glucose at these times is due to the release of epinephrine (adrenaline). You may not want to treat this high immediately, because exercise can still cause your levels to drop later.

➡ Ways to treat hypoglycemia associated with exercise include using temporary basal rates, temporarily suspending basal insulin if you continue to get low glucose levels, or ingesting extra carbohydrate without bolusing. If you do give a bolus, decrease the amount of insulin you take to cover your carbohydrate intake.

➡ If you increase your activity levels, and lose weight, you may need to change your carbohydrate ratio and/or insulin sensitivity factor (i.e., take less insulin) to avoid hypoglycemia, since you will likely be more sensitive to insulin.

CASE STUDY: MAKING CHANGES FOR EXERCISE

ALLEN

Although Allen was an "active" kind of guy, with a healthy body mass index and an A1C level between 7.0 and 7.2%, he decided to start going to the gym for weightlifting and on alternating days, for running. He consulted his health care provider, who told him to watch out for low glucose levels at the gym and to suspend his pump while running.

The first week at the gym, Allen decided to eat a small, 15-gram snack to avoid hypoglycemia. He followed a beginner's weightlifting guide (with no cardio component, such as running, cycling, rowing, etc.) and noticed the small snack seemed to cause hyperglycemia by the end of his workout over the first 2 days compared to the third day when he didn't have a snack.

	Glucose 1 hour before exercise (mg/dL)	Snack (g)	Glucose during exercise (mg/dL)	Glucose at the end exercise (mg/dL)
Day 1	89	15	130	215
Day 2	145	10	178	255
Day 3	125	0	165	178

Allen's glucose level increased because weightlifting is generally classified as anaerobic exercise, during which one's heart rate doesn't go as high as is seen in cardio-based exercises like running, cycling, rowing, or high-intensity interval training (HITT). Lifting, particularly heavy weights, puts stress on the body and can cause the release of adrenaline, cortisol, and other stress hormones that cause glucose levels to increase.

Allen talked to his health care provider and was given two options to consider: take a small amount of insulin during or immediately after his workout (such as 0.5 units in the middle of his 1-hour session) or use a temporary basal rate increase of 10% while lifting.

Allen had a very different response to running. For his first run, he didn't consume extra glucose, or decrease or suspend his basal rates. After his run, his glucose value was 130 mg/dL, but within about 20 minutes, he started to feel low. Despite 15 grams of juice and a big dinner, for which he reduced his insulin dose by 10%, at 4:00 A.M., he woke with hypoglycemia and a glucose of 57 mg/dL. His CGM showed a decrease in his glucose levels starting around 3:00 A.M., without IOB (his last bolus was 7:00 P.M. for dinner).

When doing aerobic exercise, such as running, muscles need glucose for fuel and use circulating glucose plus the glucose from glycogen stores. Muscles then need to replenish their glucose levels over the ensuing 8–48 hours, and this can cause late hypoglycemia. The timing of late hypoglycemia can vary from person to person, and with varying activity duration and intensity. If you exercise in the evening, you should be very cautious about nocturnal hypoglycemia. Minimize your risk by setting a temporary basal of 80% (or lower) for 4–6 hours when you go to sleep. If you do not have a CGM to determine how well this worked, set an alarm to wake up halfway through the night to check glucose levels and treat as needed.

Allen continued to run. Occasionally, he would take a correction dose of insulin before running if his glucose level was >180 mg/dL. However, most often and despite reducing his correction dose by 50%, he would experience a low glucose level within about 30 minutes of starting his run and would need to take oral glucose. Allen realized this was due to more effective use of insulin (faster absorption from the infusion set leading to increased muscle uptake of glucose) with exercise and having IOB from the correction dose. After talking to his health care provider, Allen decided to decrease his bolus for correction even more—by 75% so that he would take 25%—since it was so close to his run (he uses different decrease percentage depending on how close to the run he is taking insulin; 25% decrease for insulin taken 90 minutes before running, 50% decrease for insulin 60 minutes before running, and 75% decrease for insulin taken 30 minutes before his run). He also decided that if he had IOB before running, he would take oral glucose. He determined the amount of glucose he needed to ingest by thinking of what his carb ratio was at the time he started to run. When his carb ratio was 10, with 1 unit of IOB, he needed to take around 10 (or slightly more) grams of glucose to prevent hypoglycemia.

For his next run, Allen decided that the doctor had it right and that he should in fact suspend his pump during his run. He knew he would be running for 30 minutes, so he suspended for the full 30 minutes. His beginning glucose was 145 mg/dL, and his ending glucose was 90 mg/dL. About 2 hours later, though,

Allen's glucose was higher than it should have been, at 208 mg/dL. He repeated this same technique the next few runs, but each time, his CGM showed he was high 1–2 hours after the run, and he still sometimes went low during the run.

When would Allen need to suspend his pump to reduce the possibility of a low during his run and to not create a high 1–2 hours after?

Remember! You need to change your basal rate about 2 hours before to see its effect at the time you want. Many athletes suspend or decrease their insulin with a temporary basal 2 hours before their planned exercise and then resume the normal basal rate during the exercise. Some people find that they do not need a full suspension, but rather the amount of insulin they need to decrease depends on how hard they are working. A light jog may only need a 10–20% reduction while a paced run might need a 60–75% decrease. Start with a 50% reduction for the amount of time of the exercise, and start the temporary basal rate 2 hours before exercise. Decrease the amount of insulin being delivered if there is still hypoglycemia or increase the amount if glucose levels start to rise.

IN THIS CHAPTER

CHAPTER 8

THE FACTS ABOUT INFUSION SETS

There are many factors that influence which infusion set you will use when you first start the pump. You may want to see and use different infusion sets to determine which one or ones work best for you. Your choices may depend on your lifestyle and body type. (Don't forget, patch pumps do not have infusion sets.)

An infusion set consists of several components:

- **Tubing.** The tubing attaches to the insulin reservoir. The reservoir is inserted into the insulin pump, and the other end of the tubing is affixed to the insertion site itself.

- **Infusion sets and cannulas (or needles).** At the opposite end of the reservoir is the part of the infusion set that attaches to your body. It consists of an adhesive tape, a small plastic platform, and the catheter or cannula, which is a small tube that sits under the

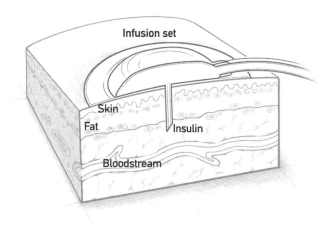

skin in the subcutaneous fat (the fat under the skin, above muscle). Through this very small tube or needle, the insulin is delivered to your body.

- **Detachable section.** There is a small platform through which the cannula connects to the tubing. A portion of the platform is detachable so that the insulin pump and tubing can be removed for activities, bathing, or other reasons. In some cases, the tubing disconnects from the infusion site near the base, and in other cases, there are a couple of inches of tubing and then a disconnect area (these can be good for young children in diapers).

For the most part, infusion sets are similar, but there are some important details that distinguish one from another and may help or hinder your diabetes care. Let's first start out with the two major categories of sets: Teflon® and metal catheters.

TYPES OF INFUSION SETS

Teflon Catheters

Teflon catheters are made of a flexible plastic material that makes them comfortable. They have one hole, or port, at the tip of the cannula to allow insulin to flow into the body's subcutaneous space. A new infusion set was designed with a second port at the side of the cannula so that if one port becomes occluded, insulin can theoretically still flow through the other port. The flexibility allows the catheter to move with you but it also can get kinked or bent while still under the skin. When this happens, insulin delivery can be slowed or stopped, potentially leading to high glucose levels. The cannula in a Teflon set comes in angles of 90° and 30°.

90° Angle

The cannula of a 90°-angle infusion set is inserted straight into the body and lies perpendicular to your skin. It can be used in any fatty area because there will be enough space between the tip of the cannula and muscle. If it is too close to the muscle, insulin absorption can be affected and sites can be more prone to kinking. For people with more fat under the skin, there is a 9-mm cannula. For leaner

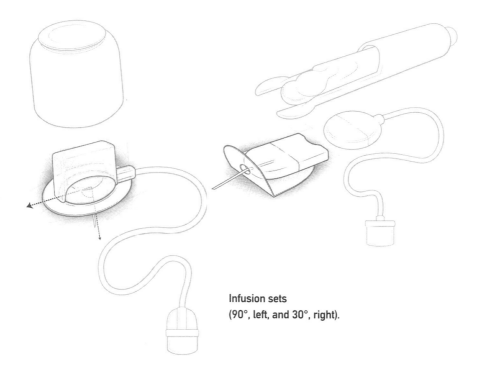

Infusion sets
(90°, left, and 30°, right).

A HANDY RULE

A good rule to think about when choosing which set to put where is if you can pinch up at least 3/4 inch or about 2 cm of fat at the site, then you can use a 90° set. However, when inserting the 90° set, it is not a good idea to pinch up the tissue. These 90° sets work very well in areas that are hard to reach (such as the upper arm, buttock, or hip) and are fleshier, or are good for people who are wary or scared of needles because there is less visibility of the needle and catheter itself. Leaner people with less body fat tend to have more problems with the 90° sets kinking or pulling free, so they might find that a 30° infusion set is a better choice.

> ## SOMETHING TO THINK ABOUT!
> Many people use either 90° or 30° sets when their infusion sets are rotated to different areas of their body. This depends on the amount of fat at each site.

people and children with less body fat, there is a 6-mm cannula. Choosing a cannula length short enough to avoid muscle but also long enough to decrease the risk of it coming out (this can be an issue with the 6-mm cannula) is important for complete and uninterrupted insulin delivery.

30° Angle
The cannula of a 30°-angle infusion set is inserted at an angle of about 30°. Because of its angled application, these sets are good for very lean or slender people without a lot of body fat. The 30° sets have a longer cannula than the 90° sets—up to 12–13 mm. These sets can be a little intimidating at first. When inserted correctly, these infusion sets avoid hitting muscle. To correctly insert this type of set, insert it at a 30° angle. If this cannula is inserted into the abdomen, the set must be inserted as close to horizontal as possible. Because of the angle and longer cannula, these sets tend to have fewer problems with kinking and pulling out, especially during exercise. It is harder to insert 30° sets in areas other than the abdominal area, but it's not impossible.

Metal Infusion Sets
Metal infusion sets, unlike the Teflon sets, have a cannula that is made of metal. They are only inserted at a 90° angle. They generally are worn with the same level of comfort as the flexible cannula. These sets are good for people who have problems with kinking or cannulas popping out. These sets have a disconnection area that is about 4 inches from the site and adhesive tape along the tubing.

Infusion Set Insertion

Infusion sets can be inserted manually or with an injector device, and some sets come with their own built-in injectors that are disposed of after inserting the infusion set. Insertion devices can sometimes help with pain or fear of the needle, since they make the process smooth and quick and often hide the needle from view. The injector devices make a clicking sound that can be intimidating for some people.

With the 30° sets, there is a small "window" area in the adhesive tape that shows where the catheter is inserted into the skin. For people who have issues with their sets falling out, this can be a useful feature because you can periodically and easily check the status or condition of your site. You can also see if there is any puffiness, redness, or other signs of a problem at the insertion site. There is no viewing window with a 90° infusion set, so the actual insertion area is less visible. A catheter on a 90° infusion set can come out without you recognizing that it has pulled away.

Inserting the 30° set manually can help people fine-tune the angle that works best for them. For both set angles, manual insertion gives the person a degree of control over pacing and placement that can't be mimicked with the insertion devices.

TUBING LENGTH

There are several lengths of tubing to connect the infusion set on the body to the reservoir in the pump. Generally, there is a shorter length (around 23–24 inches) and a longer length (about 40 inches). If the tubing length is too short, it can pull at the site and loosen the tape, leading to a kinked or removed cannula. If the tubing is too long, it has the tendency to get caught on things like doorknobs, dressers, and corners, and even on other people! Taller people tend to feel more comfortable with longer tubing, although this is not always the case.

Considerations for Tube Selection

Think about where you want to wear your pump. This placement should be the first thing to consider when determining your tubing length. Here are some other good questions to ask yourself before you choose your tubing length:

- Where will your pump be when you're sleeping? Do you want to keep it attached to you? Are you a restless sleeper or can you place your pump on your bedside table or under your pillow? Do you want to place your attached pump next to you on the bed? A longer tubing length can be more convenient for people who want to place it next to them in bed or under a pillow.

- Most people connect their pumps to their pants. Think about when you go to the bathroom and your pants are on the floor. When you stand up, is your tubing going to be long enough that it won't pull out your infusion set?

- When you change your clothing, do you need to place your pump on a nearby object, such as a dresser or bed? How close do you want to stand next to such objects?

- Some women place their pumps in carriers in their bras or on the side of their thigh under skirts or dresses. What length of tubing might this require to reach from your infusion set comfortably?

- What will you do with the extra tubing? If you prefer the longer tubing, you need to manage the excess, so it does not get caught on other things or get pulled out of your body. There are companies that make devices that roll up tubing, or you can coil it yourself and place a piece of tape around it. Just make sure that whatever approach you take, you can easily undo it so you don't accidentally pull on your set when you move your pump.

As opposed to catheter length and type, tubing length is determined by personal preference, so if you don't like the tubing length you originally chose, it's not a problem. There is plenty of variety. Tubing length is something that might also change for different activities. Keep a few different lengths on hand just in case a situation arises in which you will need longer or shorter tubing.

FACTS ABOUT INFUSION SETS

- Infusion sets are inserted at 30° or 90°, with or without an inserter (used once or multiple times).
- Infusion sets have one hole at the tip of the cannula, except one infusion set has a second hole at the side of the cannula.
- The cannula length can be 6, 8, 9, 10, 13, or 17 mm.
- The tubing length can be 18, 23, 24, 31, 32, 42, or 43 inches.
- Different companies make different lengths of tubing and cannulas that will only work with the reservoirs of certain pumps.

Priming the Infusion Set and the Cannula

Before the cannula or the needle of the infusion set is inserted into the body, the infusion set tubing has to be filled, or primed, with insulin from the reservoir that has been inserted into the pump. To assure that the tubing is filled all the way with insulin, you will observe insulin droplets coming out of the tip of the infusion set as the process to fill the tubing is completed. Because an unknown amount of insulin might leak out of the infusion set, this process can never be done while the infusion set is attached to your body.

DON'T FORGET!

Never prime, or fill, the tubing when the infusion set is attached to your body!

The cannula also needs to be filled with insulin. So once the tubing is filled to the end with insulin, and insulin is no longer dripping out of the end of the infusion set, the infusion set can be inserted. Once inserted and the needle removed, a small amount of insulin (the cannula fill amount) is delivered to fill the dead space of the cannula. The amount of insulin is programmed in the pump and is usually on the order of 0.3–0.6 units of insulin.

SITE ROTATION AND PLACEMENT OF INFUSION SET AND PUMP

It is important to understand that an infusion set is in place for 2–3 days straight. The insulin infusion and the constant presence of the catheter can cause irritation and the development of fatty lumps and scar tissue. If this occurs, absorption of insulin at that site may not be as effective. This is why site rotation (like insulin injection site rotation) is encouraged.

Creating a site-rotation plan helps eliminate the overuse or accidental reuse of a site. Some people create templates where they can record when a site was last used. Other people follow a circular rotation pattern and alternate from side to side. Your rotational preference is personal and can be changed, but make sure that you do not use the same place each time!

Where to Place Your Infusion Set

Infusion sets can be put into any area if there is enough fatty tissue to keep the cannula from pushing into muscle. Most people have some fleshy areas around their abdomen and on their buttocks. Even very thin people generally have enough tissue in these areas to successfully use an infusion set. Any 90° set can be used if there is about 3/4 inch of fat when you pinch; a 30° set takes about 1/2 inch. Your diabetes team can help you find your best places. The most common areas for site rotation are the abdomen, buttocks, upper thigh, and back of the arm. During pregnancy, the abdominal area is usually avoided.

The abdomen is the most frequently used site. Most people can use a large area of their abdomen, both above and below the waistline. Insulin is absorbed the best in this area, so it is also recommended by health care professionals. If you decide to try this area, make sure that the waistband of your clothing doesn't rub against the infusion set, since this can cause irritation and can pull the cannula free from the skin. The stomach area also offers the advantages of good visibility and easy access.

The buttocks area is also popular, particularly with young children—it is out of site and out of reach. Almost everyone has enough padding there, and a good twist around or a mirror can lead to a successful insertion. If you're wary of sitting on the infusion site, have no fear! There is plenty of space above where you actually sit that can be used for the infusion set.

The upper leg can be used, but there is more potential for hitting muscle. If you insert directly into muscle, it might be painful. In addition, it might increase the rate of absorption and cause low glucose levels.

When the back of the arm is used, the tubing must climb through your shirt and sleeves and find its way to your pump, wherever it is you intend to place it. This is something to consider when you choose tubing length.

Timing of Set Changes

Infusion sets operate best when kept in for 2–3 days. After this time period, the absorbability of the site itself diminishes. Some people see an increase in insulin resistance on or after that third day. Also,

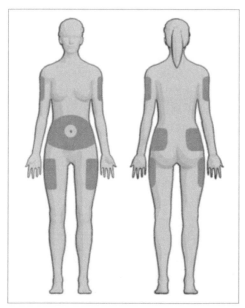

Commonly used injection sites.

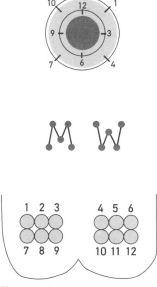

Three methods of site rotation.

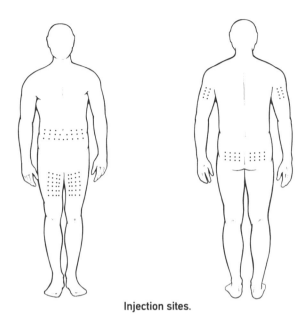

Injection sites.

if a set is left in too long, the risk of infection increases, and you certainly don't want that!

It is preferred to do a set change in the morning. This regimen gives you time to check your glucose level (blood or CGM), to be sure your new infusion set is working properly, and to check that your glucose levels are stable after the set change. If a set change is required before bed, then it is important to check glucose levels 2–3 hours later, even if this means you need to set an alarm and wake up from sleeping. Because insulin absorption can be increased after a set change, there is a risk that you might become hypoglycemic. If this routinely occurs, you might want to consider using a temporary basal rate of 70% for 4–6 hours after a set change.

Where to Place Your Pump

Where you clip, hang, bag, or store your insulin pump is up to you (unless you're using a patch pump). There are some common ways to carry it and some rather creative ways to deal with its constant presence.

It is easiest to wear the pump around your waist. You can put it in your pocket or clip it onto your belt or waistband (pumps come with clips and holders). In addition, you can buy pouches and cases with belt loops and clips. Some children need to be kept away from their pumps, so harnesses and pouches are good options (these also keep the pump away from curious classmates and friends who might want to press buttons). If you keep your pump in your front pocket (this is often more possible for men with looser pants), then you might think about clipping a small hole in the inside of the pocket, so you can feed your tubing through the hole—the tubing will have less opportunity to get caught on something. When wearing skirts or dresses without pockets or waistbands, some women use pouches and similar devices to strap their pumps to the inside of their thighs (like garters with a pouch), they put their pump in the top of a knee-high or tall boot, or they clip the pump to their bras.

There are other situations when you will have to deal with the placement of your pump that might not occur to you until you encounter them, but below are a few to think about.

Sleeping

If you are a restless sleeper, it might be a good idea to find a way to attach the pump comfortably to your pajamas. Or try placing it under your pillow (but be aware that you might not hear the alarms). If you sleep fairly calmly, you can put it on a bedside table or next to you in the bed. (If you have a restless partner in bed with you, then you might want to think about the possibility of him or her rolling over it as well.)

Many people worry about rolling over their infusion site, tubing, and pump while sleeping, but everything is durable and should survive the impact. You shouldn't be able to feel the infusion site when you roll onto it (if there is tenderness or pain, then there might be something wrong with the site, and a site rotation might be necessary). Tubing shouldn't kink, and it takes a significant amount of direct pressure to the buttons to activate them. The amount of pressure from your body is spread out when you are lying down, and there is plenty of give in your mattress to avoid any kinking or unwanted pump-button activation.

Exercise

Most pumps are fairly sturdy and water resistant, so you can wear one during exercise—regardless of sweating. A number of protective hard cases are available if you don't want to remove your pump during rougher sports (such cases are highly recommended). Also, activities that involve water (e.g., swimming, scuba diving, snorkeling, water skiing, tubing, or surfing) might require you to disconnect the pump. You need to know if the pump you are using is waterproof or not. Most pumps are water resistant and can get wet, but you might want to be more cautious when submerging them in water. Even if the pump is designed to be water resistant or waterproof, if there is any small crack in the casing, this could ruin your pump or cause a dangerous malfunction.

When you disconnect from the pump, the cannula is left inserted into your body and the tubing and pump are removed. Often, sets will come with clips or coverings to keep the site clean and free of things like sand. The sets are designed so only insulin via the tubing is allowed into your body, so don't worry about swimming with a disconnected set. When you disconnect for sports and exercise, it is important to watch your blood glucose carefully and to periodically reconnect to give a small amount of insulin to counteract the loss of your basal insulin.

A NOTE ABOUT DISCONNECTING YOUR PUMP

It is a good idea to suspend your pump's functions when you disconnect. When doing this, your pump will stop delivering insulin, and the pump will not account for insulin you did not receive. When most pumps are suspended, they sound an alarm every half hour or so to remind you that it has been suspended. This alarm will notify you if you happen to fall asleep without reconnecting or forget that you are in the suspend mode.

Intimacy

When you are engaged in intimate activities, pumps can easily be disconnected and put away. Just don't forget to put your pump on after.

Showers and Baths

You need to know if your pump is water resistant or waterproof. If it is not waterproof, you should disconnect from the pump for showers and baths (and swimming and hot tubs). Remember to reconnect after you are done. The pumps that are water resistant or waterproof can be worn in the shower and the bath, although most people disconnect for bathing anyway.

Remove your pump if you are going into a hot tub or Jacuzzi. The pump may be waterproof, but the water may be warm enough to spoil insulin.

TROUBLESHOOTING ISSUES AT THE INSERTION SITE

Here are some common issues that you might experience with your infusion sets (or patch pump):

- **Irritation from the tape.** Some people have issues with the adhesive on the tapes irritating their skin, lasting too long, or coming off early. Although allergies and sensitivities are uncommon, they do unfortunately happen. Some people experience a rash after removing the tape or while the set is inserted into the area. There are several wipes that can add a level of protection between the skin and the adhesive. In addition, a spray of a nasal allergy medication, fluticasone propionate (a corticosteroid), may decrease irritation from allergy when sprayed onto the skin and allowed to dry before insertion of the infusion set. If that is not enough, inserting the set through a small hole in a hypoallergenic dressing placed on the skin before the infusion set also helps completely separate the irritant from the skin.

- **Adhesive on the skin.** If you have problems with tape staying on (this is very common), there are several wipes that will help with adhesion. It is important to always start by wiping the intended area with alcohol. This step helps remove bacteria and surface oils, which can impede the stickiness of the tape (on the note of bacteria, don't blow on your site to dry it because this can introduce germs to the area and increase the chances of getting an infection). If you need even more assistance with getting the tape to stay attached to your skin, you can try more potent preparations. The only problem with some of these potent wipes is removing the set later. People who sweat a lot or exercise frequently might also try placing another piece of tape over the top of the set. You might also think about putting a piece of tape about 2 inches above the site for added security in case tubing is caught on something. Doing this is especially helpful if you have trouble with the set sticking in place.

If you have a problem with removal, then there are products that can help with that too (they've thought of everything!). All of these products can be applied to the top of the tape and then left for a few minutes to sink in and start to dissolve the stickiness underneath. Then as you slowly remove the tape, wipe the solvent under the tape to detach the rest of it. Just make sure you wash off the solvent completely, or your next set might not stick very well.

- **Bubbles in tubing.** Several things can cause bubbles to appear in your tubing, and it is important to regularly check for these because an inch of air in the tubing can be equivalent to half a unit of insulin! For many people, that can be a significant amount of their basal rate and can cause a high glucose level. Bubbles can form from insulin going from cold to room temperature (this applies to people who take their insulin bottles right from the refrigerator before filling the reservoir). If you can, try to let your insulin warm up a little bit before filling your reservoir and before changing your set. A change in altitude, such as when flying in an airplane or driving into the mountains, can increase bubble frequency. This scenario can happen in a patch pump, too, but there is no way to check for bubbles, since you cannot see inside the pod. Be sure to check glucose levels frequently or watch your CGM closely to determine if you had bubbles due to altitude changes.

Bubbles can be removed by a Fill or Prime function. The pump records this amount of insulin but does not count it toward a meal or correction bolus, so the pump won't think that there is active insulin. Make sure you disconnect before you prime to remove bubbles, or you might receive extra insulin that you don't need. It's a worthwhile habit to check for bubbles in the morning and before you go to bed. Bubbles, other than keeping you from receiving insulin, will not harm you if they enter your body.

- **Pain.** If your set is painful, it might be a sign of infection or that you have inserted your cannula too close to muscle. In either case, it is a good idea to change your set because insulin absorption will be affected and will be absorbed faster or not at all, depending on what's wrong. If there is any puffiness, redness, swelling, discharge, or warmth at your set, you should change your set and then monitor your glucose levels as well as your body temperature. If you develop a fever, it could mean that you have an infection, and you should not only change your set immediately but also contact your health care team or your primary care physician. Without a fever, it is most likely okay to just change your set. However, if you have a painful, red, hot lump—which might contain bacteria and pus—that gets worse or won't go away, you should contact your health care team.

WHEN DO YOU CONTACT YOUR HEALTH CARE TEAM ABOUT AN INFECTED SET?

- If you have a fever >99.9° F
- If the site is hot, hard, and red and the size of the redness grows over a day. Check this by drawing a circle the size of the redness with a permanent marker. If the redness spreads past the original circle, call your health care team. You will likely be prescribed an antibiotic to threat the infection and also local measures, such as hot soaks.

- **High blood glucose after a set change.** If your blood glucose level increases (without an obvious cause) after a set change, you might have forgotten to prime or fill your cannula. This prime is different from the prime or fill that fills the tubing with insulin. The cannula cannot be filled until after the needle (in the case of the Teflon sets) has been removed after an insertion, and until you have connected the now primed tubing to the infusion set.

Taking proper care of your site by cleaning it thoroughly before insertion, checking regularly for bubbles, and changing it on time will help prevent highs and infections from happening.

ON THE HORIZON

The goal is to improve infusion sets so they fail less often and last longer. For individuals wearing pumps and CGM, another goal is to integrate in the sensor and the infusion set, so there is one insertion site on the body. There is an infusion with two holes, or ports, for insulin delivery. There is research assessing strategies to extend infusion set wear to a week, or maybe even longer. There is the concept that insulin might be modified so that the insulin doesn't form fibrils that likely lead to early infusion set clogging and failure. And there have been prototypes of combined infusion set and CGM; but for this to be a realistic option, infusion sets need to last as long as CGM devices—a week or more.

CHAPTER REVIEW

➡ The infusion set is made up of tubing that attaches at one end to the insulin reservoir in the insulin pump. The other end affixes to the insertion site itself—the cannula or needle and the detachable section.

➡ There are several lengths of tubing to connect the infusion set on the body to the reservoir in the pump. Determining the correct length(s) for you (from 23–24 inches to about 40 inches) is important.

➡ It is important to understand that an infusion set is in place for 2–3 days straight. Local insulin infusion and the constant presence of the catheter can cause irritation and the development of fatty lumps and scar tissue. If this occurs, absorption of insulin at that site may not work as expected. This is why site rotation is encouraged.

➡ Issues that occur, such as irritation at the insertion site, residual adhesive on the skin, bubbles in the tubing, pain at the insertion site, and high glucose levels after insertion, require troubleshooting.

➡ Don't forget: never prime the tubing if the infusion set is connected to your body.

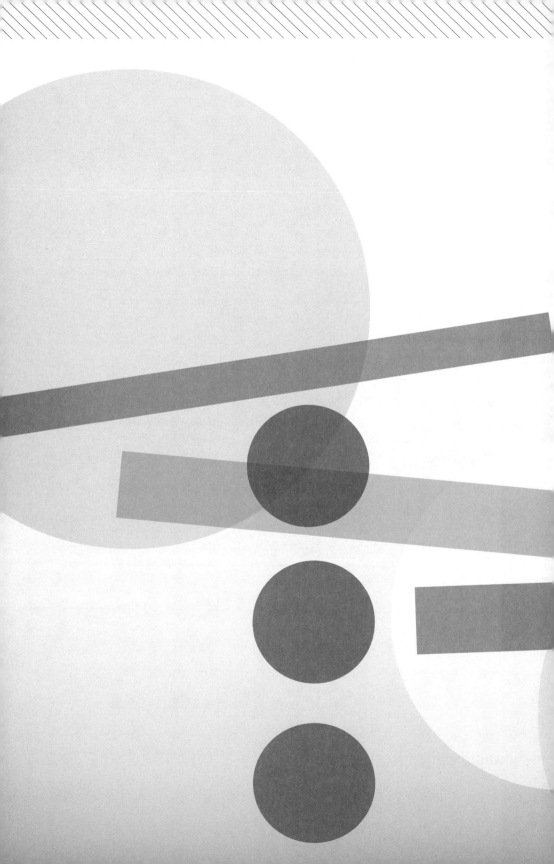

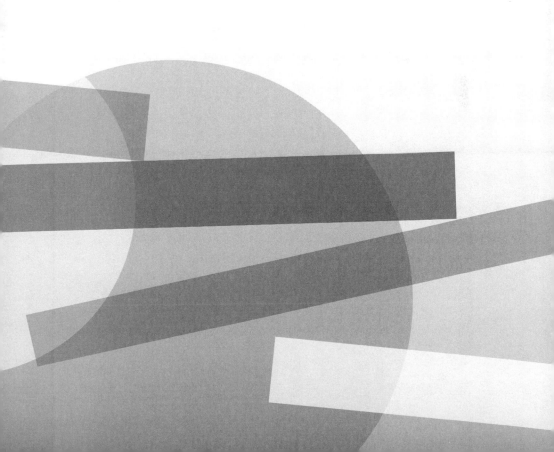

SECTION 3:

UPLOADS, CGM, AND CLOSING THE LOOP

IN THIS CHAPTER

➡ How to Upload Your Pump or CGM

➡ What Downloads Can Look Like

➡ How to Interpret Data

➡ At Your Diabetes Appointment

CHAPTER 9

UPLOADING PUMPS AND CGM FOR INTERPRETATION

Essentially, each pump, sensor, and continuous glucose monitor (CGM) company has a version of software, and each of these versions is slightly different from the other. As a result, in 2013, recommendations for standardizing glucose reports were proposed so that there is a universal reporting system for all devices to replace or augment what is currently available. At the writing of this second edition, many companies plan to continue to have their individual reporting systems and plan to include a universal report if one becomes available.

HOW TO UPLOAD YOUR PUMP OR CGM

Check to see how your device(s) uploads. You may need a cable, or use the glucose meter or an upload device that serves as a wireless conduit for data transfer.

Pump and CGM combination systems will automatically upload all data into one program and display the information in the same graphs and pictures. If you use a pump and CGM from different companies, you may need to download two separate reports from different software/websites, unless you can find a universal software/website that accepts upload from multiple systems or devices and download them into one comprehensive report. There are several websites that offer this and show data differently. If your devices are compatible, the different websites show data in various colors and formats so that you can choose which ones make most sense to you. Below, the various types of reports and how to interpret them are highlighted.

Some CGMs now transmit data directly to an app on a cell phone. These are real-time data, and you can review your reports through the app. This app can upload your information directly to the corresponding software/website for viewing your data (which often has an app as well). This process makes it easy to view data frequently and assess for patterns and trends and how to change settings to improve glucose management.

Be sure to click through all the different report types provided by your program(s). One way of displaying data may make more sense to you than another and help you see where you need to make setting changes. Again, the more often you upload and review data, the more familiar you will become with how these reports can help you manage your diabetes.

WHAT DOWNLOADS CAN LOOK LIKE

There are several ways to look at your pump, glucose meter, and CGM data. These include a logbook, trend graphs, pie charts, and data tables. The logbook is just a digital version of a handwritten log. Trend graphs, pie charts, and data tables are visual representations of the logbook information that make it easier to spot patterns and trends. The trend graphs and pie charts are colorful visual representations of your glucose numbers, averages, and high/low patterns, whereas the data table contains just numbers and values. Each method of displaying your information can be reviewed to identify specific problems or times of good control.

HOW TO INTERPRET DATA

Colors
Many software programs use different colors to facilitate spotting patterns. In most systems, color coding is used to indicate data above, within, and below the target range in logbooks, pie charts, and trend graphs, as well as in other reports.

Logbooks

Logbooks, like the paper ones you might have been given when you were first diagnosed, are grids containing all of the pertinent information that affects your diabetes. They are either very detailed, or they can just display your glucose values at certain times of day (before or after meals). Blood glucose meter and CGM data can also be uploaded into a logbook format.

Trend Graphs

A trend graph is often the first thing that your diabetes team will look at because they easily show many days of data laid over each other. A trend graph has your blood or sensor glucose values along the vertical axis and the time of day along the horizontal axis. The horizontal axis generally shows 24 hours and can start at either 5:00 A.M. or midnight, depending on which pump, CGM, or meter you use. Customizable target ranges can be set and are shown as a shaded horizontal bar through the whole graph. Multiple days are represented on the graph as different colored lines with small symbols at each blood glucose value. On a CGM graph, the colored lines are more fluid, with no individual symbols because there are many, many more data points. There is usually also a dotted or bolded line that runs through the graph as the running average of all the days' values.

Trend graphs make it easy to spot repeating patterns. Trend graphs are also helpful because you can see your highest and lowest

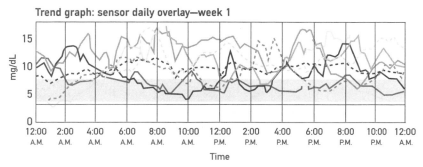

Trend graph: sensor daily overlay—week 1

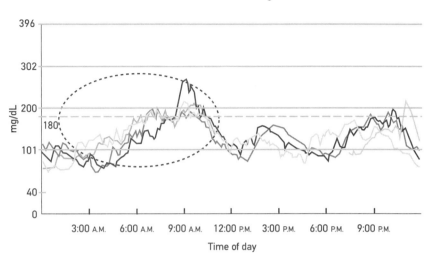

Effect of Dawn Phenomenon on Morning Blood Glucose

values on the graph, and with the adjustable target range, you can also see how often your values swing outside this range.

The graph generated by a CGM shows a spike of numbers beginning around 4:00 A.M. This graph offers a good visualization of the dawn phenomenon (it is circled in the graph above). The dawn phenomenon occurs when certain hormone levels, such as cortisol and growth hormone, spike in the early morning hours, resulting in increased glucose levels, which in turn requires a higher insulin dosage. Looking at this graph will help you identify the dawn phenomenon and allow you to treat it by increasing your early morning basal rate.

Pie Charts

Pie charts show the averages for the numbers in your target range, above it, and below it. Each pie chart represents a different time of day (e.g., before and after breakfast) or a specific day. Generally, each section is a different color, making it easy to see that a majority of your values are in a certain range. Ideally, you should aim for as much time in the target range as possible, but many people have difficulty achieving more than 50–60% of the time in that range. Similarly, you should aim for as little time in the hypoglycemia range as possible. Many people have difficulty achieving <11% of their values in the low glucose range.

Although pie charts identify times when there are too many values in the high or low range, they don't show you the most extreme values. As a result, data can also be displayed as a bar with percent in the very low range, low range, target range, high range, and very high range. Some display formats use the dangerously high and low ranges as an additional analysis.

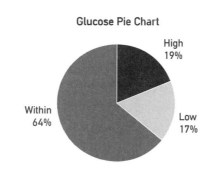

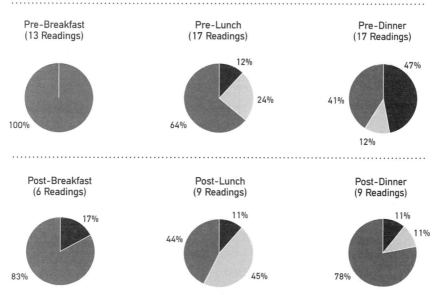

Data Tables

Data tables are grids of numbers, including highest and lowest numbers, standard deviation (which is a measure of glycemic variability), averages, number of times glucose testing was performed, frequency of infusion set changes, and percentage above and below target during the days you've selected for review. These types of tables work better with more data points and therefore are optimized when CGM is used.

Average Numbers

Average numbers are used to determine glucose levels during specific times of day, such as when you first wake up or when you go to sleep. Averages don't show the highest or lowest numbers (for example, after lunch for the past 2 weeks).

Standard Deviation

The standard deviation (abbreviated SD) assesses how frequently and how far you go above or below your average glucose value. The standard deviation is a reflection of the typical excursion or increment, above or below, your average blood glucose or your average sensor glucose value. Optimally, the standard deviation should be as small as possible. Because the standard deviation reflects the degree of variability of your glucose numbers, it is not beneficial to have a high standard deviation.

Percent (%) High, Low, and in Range

The data sheet also shows the percentage (%) of glucose values in the high, low, and target range, just like the pie charts, but these are numerical values rather than graphic representations. These data can be used like the pie charts, and target ranges can be customized for each individual.

AT YOUR DIABETES APPOINTMENT

When you see your health care team, team members should download the information from your pump, glucose meter, and CGM at

These are two displays from the 2013 published report of a consensus panel of endocrinologists who proposed a standardized way of reporting sensor glucose data from device uploads.

Glucose values that have been obtained fall either in target, or above or below target. These data reveal that dangerously high and low values put you at risk for severe hypoglycemia or diabetic ketoacidosis.

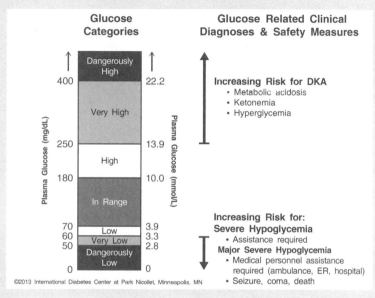

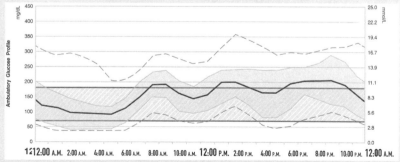

In addition, they use a sensor glucose display that shows the median sensor glucose values by time, with the blue shaded area showing where 50% of sensor glucose values lie from the 25th to 75th percentile for glucose data. The dotted lines represent the 10th and 90th percentile glucose ranges.

the clinic, or they may ask you to bring in your own downloaded data. With these tools, they can help you identify areas of optimal and less-than-optimal glucose control and help you determine a course of action. While a lot of focus goes into areas of improvement, it is just as important to celebrate when you have good averages, low standard deviations, and lots of in-range values.

Ultimately, the more you review your data, the better your diabetes control should be. Regularly uploading and reviewing the information stored in your pump and CGM will enable you to make changes in your pump settings and diabetes regimen at your health care visits and during the months in between.

CHAPTER REVIEW

➡ The value of looking at your data—at home and during your clinic visit—is immense. Assessing your data between clinic visits should help you understand if you are achieving your glucose goals. It is most important for you to go over your uploads during your clinic visits, particularly in relation to your recently obtained A1C value. If you are not where you desire to be, discuss your data with your health care provider to determine what changes need to be made.

➡ Learn the different reports and decide which ones help you the most. The digital version of the logbook looks very similar to what you kept when you first were diagnosed with diabetes. Trend graphs, pie charts, and data tables may take you longer to learn to use, but they have the ability for you to see emerging areas of concern with your diabetes control, as well as areas in which you are in target most of the time.

➡ Look at patterns and trends and at your behaviors, the number of boluses, and the number of glucose measurements, and keep making progress. With all the data generated by your insulin and your CGM, you and your health care provider cannot miss the opportunity to make changes in your regimen that are data driven and supported.

IN THIS CHAPTER

CHAPTER 10

THE FACTS ABOUT CONTINUOUS GLUCOSE MONITORING

TYPES OF CONTINUOUS GLUCOSE MONITORING: RETROSPECTIVE AND REAL-TIME

There are two types of continuous glucose monitors (CGMs): retrospective (or diagnostic or blinded) and real-time. Retrospective CGMs belong to your doctor's office. They are used infrequently (one, two, or three times a year). While you are wearing a retrospective CGM, you do not see the glucose data from the sensor displayed on a monitor or screen. Instead, when the sensor wear is over, the recorder or monitor is uploaded into a computer program that displays graphs, charts, and tables of your sensor glucose data. These data can then be merged with a written log or an app of your activity, food intake, and medication to give you and your diabetes team a picture of how your diabetes therapy and lifestyle affect your glucose levels. Although retrospective continuous glucose monitoring is used more by people with type 2 diabetes, some people with type 1 diabetes use retrospective continuous glucose monitoring as well. In type 1 diabetes, it is particularly useful to obtain a detailed profile of glucose patterns and trends and examine nighttime glucose levels, uncover unexpected hypoglycemia, assess postmeal glucose excursions, and determine if there is the dawn phenomenon. This way, you can determine if your insulin regimen is optimal or if you need to consider making a change in insulin dosages or in the number of injections. You may also need to consider switching from multiple daily injections (MDI) to an insulin pump, or the other way around.

HOW REAL-TIME CONTINUOUS GLUCOSE MONITORING WORKS AND ITS COMPONENTS

Real-time CGMs are owned by you, and these devices allow you to see your glucose levels and trends continuously. Starting to use a real-time CGM is similar to starting an insulin pump. It takes knowledge, training, motivation, and support from others. A CGM provides a lot of additional information about your glucose levels. It checks your glucose numerous times—up to 255 times—per day and can signal an alert if your levels are outside, or predicted to be outside, of your target range, or if they are increasing or decreasing too rapidly. A CGM can send data directly to a monitor/receiver or to a remote device such as a phone or a watch, and it can generate trend graphs through uploading into computer programs for later analysis. In certain newer pump systems, CGM data can stop insulin delivery at a set threshold or at a predicted threshold and also allow for the delivery of basal insulin based on automated insulin delivery algorithms in hybrid closed-loop systems. As you can see, a CGM provides a lot of information and potentially automation, but for it to be helpful, you need to know how to use it and how to interpret the information it generates. Then, with the help of your diabetes team, you can turn the information, data, and automation into action to improve your diabetes care and outcomes.

A CGM continuously measures the glucose level in the fluid under your skin (your interstitial glucose level, which is usually very close to your blood glucose level) and reports a new value every 5 minutes all day and all night. This method produces far more information than normal self-monitoring of blood glucose (SMBG).

Continuous glucose monitoring measures glucose in the interstitial space that contains the fluid that surrounds your body's cells. Glucose enters the interstitial tissue as it works its way to your cells, where it can be used for energy. Because a CGM measures glucose in the interstitial fluid and not the blood, values obtained at the same time from SMBG and from a CGM may not be exactly identical. This result is particularly true when the glucose level is rapidly changing, such as right after a meal or during exercise. For this rea-

OTHER SENSOR GLUCOSE DEVICES

A new type of glucose monitoring system has been developed that doesn't display all of the information continuously, but can be swiped (usually four, six, eight, or more times per day) with a reader to show the glucose level at that time. Data can be downloaded from the device to get a more comprehensive picture of glucose trends and patterns. The device measures interstitial glucose and is worn subcutaneously (under the skin) for up to 14 days. This device does not work like other CGMs, since it will not alert or sound an alarm when glucose falls or rises out of the target range. This device does not need to be calibrated with a fingerstick blood glucose measurement.

son, the real-time numbers displayed on a CGM receiver are actually about 10–20 minutes behind the reading of blood glucose. Depending on rate of change in blood glucose levels, the CGM values are generally within 20% of the blood glucose number. At the time of the writing of this second edition, some systems continue to require confirmation of CGM glucose with a blood glucose fingerstick measurement before dosing insulin, while others do not. The CGM devices approved by the U.S. Food and Drug Administration not requiring SMBG confirmation allow insulin to be given to correct a high glucose or to treat a low glucose level based on the CGM value itself—but only if there is matching of the CGM glucose level with symptoms and there is confidence that the CGM is working well. Because CGMs have become more accurate and are allowed to automate insulin delivery in the first hybrid closed-loop systems available, in future devices, it is likely that there will no longer be a need to confirm CGM readings with blood glucose measurements.

Basic Components

The three parts of the real-time CGM system are the sensor, the transmitter, and the receiver/monitor. In one system, the receiver/monitor can be a cell phone. Another new system, still being studied at the writing of the second edition, is implanted for 3–6 months, and a receiver is worn over the sensor insertion site.

Overall, the components communicate with each other to provide you with the glucose level in your interstitial fluid. You can get information in real time by looking at the receiver/monitor or phone, or by looking at a secondary screen such as a watch or tablet. You can get alerts to warn of actual or predicted high and low glucose levels, and rapidly changing glucose levels. You can review retrospective data by uploading the CGM to a computer program or by having information sent automatically to the "cloud," where the data are stored and retrieved for display. Each separate part of the system is critically important for its functioning.

The Sensor

The sensor sits under the skin and is similar in size and shape to an infusion set cannula. The sensor is inserted with the help of a needle (which is removed after insertion) and an inserter. It is made of a flexible fiber-plastic material that reacts to glucose changes and sends the information to the transmitter. Once inserted, the sensor should be unnoticed and painless. Different sensors have different lengths, between 12 and 15 mm (1/2 to 3/4 inch), and are injected at either a 45° or 90° angle. They last between 3 and 7 days. While sensors read interstitial glucose continuously, the devices display a glucose reading every 5 minutes while you are wearing them. When you first insert the sensor, it takes time to get the sensor in contact with enough interstitial fluid for it to start measuring glucose levels. During this "warm-up" time, the sensor does not send glucose values to the transmitter and you will not see any values on the CGM receiver screen. Although it varies depending on which device you use, this warm-up period is generally 2 hours.

On the outside, the sensor resembles an infusion set—it has a plastic top covering the sensor and is held to the skin with an adhesive. The transmitter is connected to this plastic part. The first sensors generally needed to be replaced after 3 days, but advances in sensor development now have sensors lasting 6–7 days, with the hope that soon they will last between 10 and 14 days.

The sensor can be placed in a variety of places on your body, including arms, legs, abdomen, or buttocks. You need enough body

WHAT'S UP NEXT FOR SENSORS?

Implanted sensors are now being developed. These sensors are implanted under the skin and can last 3 months (there are hopes that they will ultimately last even longer than that). They are not connected to any device on the surface of the skin, but have a receiver placed over them that is held in place with straps.

fat to accommodate a sensor. A good rule for this is, if you can pinch up enough body fat with two fingers to be able to insert a sensor, then that's a good location. If you are someone who does not have many areas with a lot of body fat, you might need to consider the different insertion angles and sensor lengths when choosing a CGM. Another thing to consider is that these are the same areas where infusion sets are worn. There must be at least 2 inches between the infusion set and a sensor. Sensors might not function well in areas that have swollen tissue from repeated insulin administration. Research is being done to enable the infusion set and the CGM to be placed on a single platform, so this rule will likely change in the future.

The Transmitter

The transmitter sends information from the sensor to the monitor/receiver. It clips into the plastic head of the sensor platform, either on top or on the side, and is generally taped down after the connection. Radio wave or Bluetooth technology sends the readings to the receiver. Depending on the brand, the transmitter can communicate with a monitor/receiver that is between 6 and 20 feet away. Sometimes, the signal can be blocked or interrupted by cell phones or other transmitting frequencies, but the signal will be restored automatically once the source of the interruption is removed. Transmitters vary in size (6–12 mm or 1/4–1/2 inch in height) and shape; some are rectangular and some are round.

Transmitters have batteries that need to be replaced or recharged regularly. Transmitters with batteries that need recharging usually have battery lives that last through several sensors, and the status of the transmitter battery can be viewed on the receiver. All transmitters are waterproof, so you can shower, bathe, or swim without worrying that they will become damaged. If you are swimming, especially in the ocean, you must make sure the transmitters and sensors are securely adhered to your body so you don't lose them. Although most systems are waterproof, data do not transmit well through water, so the sensor signal may be lost.

The Receiver/Monitor

This is the part of the CGM that displays the current sensor glucose level as well as trend arrows, graphs, and device information, such as battery life, transmitter signal strength, date, and time. There are different styles of receivers. Some use the same screen as your insulin pump, some are small handheld devices, and others can transmit to your smartphone and to your specialized watch via the phone so you don't have to carry another device. Handheld receivers can be kept in your pocket, purse, or elsewhere nearby. Real-time CGM systems have alarms to warn you of high and low sensor glucose levels.

There are alarms that tell you when you need to calibrate your system and some can tell you when your glucose levels are rising or falling too fast. Alarms will notify you when your receiver or transmitter battery is running low or when the signal from the transmitter is lost. Like a cell phone, most receivers let you choose between a sound and a vibrating alert. All receivers also have a backlight, so information can be viewed in the dark.

MISCONCEPTIONS ABOUT CONTINUOUS GLUCOSE MONITORING

CGM Levels and Blood Glucose Levels Are Identical

There is a 10- to 20-minute lag between the glucose levels obtained with a CGM and those obtained with SMBG. But even with this, the CGM values are generally within 20% of the SMBG levels.

Sensors Can Be Worn Infrequently

If you wear the real-time sensor for only a couple days a month, you may not see the same benefits as someone who wears it continuously. The Sensor-Augmented Pump Therapy for A1C Reduction (STAR) 3 study (described in Chapter 1) showed that when someone wore a CGM for about 60% of the time, A1C was lowered by 0.5%, but when a CGM was worn for 80–100% of the time, there was a 1.2% drop in A1C. If you don't want to use a CGM all of the time, consider using it during illnesses, when glucose management is not optimal; while traveling; after you change your insulin dosages, your diet, or other parts of your regimen; or when you change your usual schedule. It may help you better manage your diabetes during these times.

Continuous Glucose Monitoring Can Be Kept Private

Using and reviewing the data from a CGM can lead to success, but keeping up with all that data will make it hard to keep your CGM a secret. If your transmitter is visible or you are going to look at the monitor frequently (there might be the option of looking on your phone or your watch), respond to the alerts, and alter your regimen, people will likely see you using it or doing something to manage your diabetes. Like the pump, there is no reason to advertise or conceal this important device. If strangers see it, you might want to stop questions by giving an explanation—or have an answer ready if they ask. It is best to have the support of friends and family, because it will make using the CGM and managing your diabetes easier.

Using a CGM Can Cause Information Overload

Because a real-time CGM gives a lot of information—hundreds of glucose values per day—it takes time to determine how to use the numbers, alerts, and trends to best manage your diabetes. Working with your diabetes team is necessary at the beginning, but as time goes on, you will gain expertise and experience. Many of the alarms can be turned off to avoid information overload, and only the ones that you and your doctor deem important can be enabled. Once you feel like you have a good grasp on your alarms and glucose levels, adding in more alarms and alerts can help you tighten your control. Alarm fatigue is a real thing, so make sure you turn on a realistic amount of alarms so that you continue to use the CGM. As discussed above, partial use of a CGM is not as helpful as use 80–100% of the time. *Don't forget: the stand-alone CGMs have a lower alarm at 50 or 55 mg/dL that cannot be turned off for safety reasons.*

There Is No Room on Your Body for Both a CGM and an Insulin Pump

You have enough places on your body for a CGM and an insulin pump. The sensors are about the size of a pump infusion site and must be placed at least 2 inches from a pump site. You rotate the sites like you do with your pump and can use any body area where you can pinch up enough skin with two fingers. Even very young children can use a CGM with pumps. Generally, this results in a CGM on one buttock cheek and the infusion set on the other. This setup does require some careful planning and rotation. However, very young and very small children have used and do use CGMs and insulin pumps together successfully.

A CGM Must Be Used with an Insulin Pump

Although CGM and pump therapies work well together, there are many people on MDI therapy who successfully use the CGM to help manage their diabetes.

APPROPRIATE CANDIDATES FOR CONTINUOUS GLUCOSE MONITORING

A CGM should be considered for anyone with type 1 diabetes. And there is no reason to wait to get a CGM; right at diagnosis is as good a time as any. But you are a particularly good candidate if you are experiencing wide fluctuations in glucose levels; are having frequent, severe, unrecognized, or nocturnal hypoglycemia; have trouble with glucose control during exercise or periods of stress; have not achieved your target A1C; or want more data to further improve your journey with diabetes. In addition, it is important to consider the following issues:

Willingness to Wear a Sensor

If you are going to start using a CGM, you need to know that you will have a sensor and a transmitter constantly attached to you. You might want to tape a transmitter to your skin to see what it is like to have a sensor.

A Good Support System

Like most aspects of diabetes, going it alone is not the best approach. Having your parents, family members, spouse, and friends involved can help you learn how and where to insert sensors, how to trouble-shoot problems, and how to best use the information generated by the CGM. With support, your likelihood of success increases.

A Diabetes Team Familiar with the CGM

You need a knowledgeable and accessible diabetes team that is experienced in teaching you how to get the best outcomes out of a CGM.

Willingness to Change

The information obtained with a CGM might indicate that you need to make significant changes to your diabetes regimen. You must be open to these changes to make a CGM worthwhile. CGMs are useful when you are willing to upload and review the numbers regularly as well as watching in real time.

Skin That Can Tolerate Continuous Glucose Monitoring

You will need to use adhesive to secure the sensor and transmitter. It might take some time finding the best way to secure the devices, and make sure you give the body areas you use time to heal between insertions.

Cost of Continuous Glucose Monitoring

Health insurance coverage and the cost of a CGM must be taken into consideration. If your insurance does cover a CGM, you still might have a large co-pay. Insurance will not likely cover a CGM for type 2 diabetes. Medicare will only cover if confirmatory finger-sticks are not required. Be sure that you are able to bear the cost of a CGM before you decide to purchase and use one.

EXCITING NEWS ABOUT CONTINUOUS GLUCOSE MONITORING

At the time of the writing of this second edition, the reliability and safety of dosing insulin and making other treatment decisions based on CGM values without a confirmatory fingerstick have been deter-mined for one CGM system. In addition, a CGM can be used to dose basal insulin in new automated insulin delivery systems, referred to as hybrid closed-loop devices. However, it is still recommended to test blood glucose levels to verify the accuracy of the sensor values if symptoms don't match CGM glucose levels or there is any ques-tion about sensor functioning. In addition, CGM systems need to have the sensor calibrated at least two or more times a day to assure sensor accuracy.

CHAPTER REVIEW

➡ Use a CGM if you want the extra information the glucose sensor provides. It gives hundreds of glucose values per day, alerts you if glucose values are outside or predicted to be outside your target range or are changing rapidly, shows trend graphs, and can upload data to computer programs for later analysis. For a CGM to help improve diabetes care, you need to know what to do with all the additional information and how to use it in collaboration with your diabetes team.

➡ There are many common misconceptions about continuous glucose monitor-ing. You must understand that a CGM gives a lot of information and that the simultaneous values for a CGM and SMBG might be different because of the different conditions under which the glucose levels are measured.

➡ Continuous glucose monitoring should be considered if you are experiencing wide fluctuations in glucose levels; are having frequent, severe, unrecognized, or nocturnal hypoglycemia; have trouble with glucose control during exercise or periods of stress; have not achieved your target A1C; or want more information for your journey with diabetes.

➡ There are a few different CGM systems available in the U.S. market. You should discuss which system you want with your diabetes team and with friends who are already using a CGM. Do your research, too. Visit the CGM manufacturer websites. You might also want to check the Diabetes Forecast consumer guide. To make the best decisions regarding your diabetes, you need to have information to make the right choice for you. The major differences among CGM devices are in whether fingersticks are required when making treatment decisions, the size and insertion angle of the sensors, how long the sensors last, whether the monitor is separate or integrated with an insulin pump or can transmit to a phone, the look and feel of the sensor inserter, range, meter compatibility, transmitter and receiver battery type and lifespan, what alerts are available, and what is displayed on the monitor with regard to arrows, trend graphs, and other numbers.

➡ Only one CGM is currently approved for use in treatment-based decisions; others are not. Make sure to continue to check glucose levels and calibrate your CGM system. Check with the manufacturing company if you are unsure if your device is approved to dose insulin and treat hypoglycemia without a confirming SMBG level.

IN THIS CHAPTER

➡ How to Use Trend Arrows, Alarms, Alerts, and Graphs

➡ What's Involved with Wearing a CGM?

➡ Tips for Taping and Keeping Your Sensor On

CHAPTER 11

HOW TO USE REAL-TIME CONTINUOUS GLUCOSE MONITORING AND CGM DATA

HOW TO USE TREND ARROWS, ALARMS, ALERTS, AND GRAPHS

The receiver of a continuous glucose monitor (CGM) gives you a lot of information, such as trend arrows, alerts, and alarms. You must know how to read and understand these parts to benefit from a CGM and the information it generates.

Trend Arrows
Trend arrows tell you if your glucose levels are stable, rising or falling moderately (1–2 mg/dL per minute), or rising or falling quickly (>2 mg/dL per minute). Different systems have different designs for these arrows, but they all essentially display the same information: the rate of change of glucose levels and the direction in which they are going. Trend arrows can be used to adjust your diabetes management plan. When combined with the current glucose value shown on a CGM, trend arrows will give you a forecast of your glucose levels, just like a weather forecast. If your current level is within your target range but the trend arrows indicate that your levels are rising or falling rapidly, you will know to take action to prevent anything from actually happening. These actions could include issuing a correction bolus from your pump (for highs) or taking some glucose tabs or adjusting your basal rate (for lows). Similarly, if you are about to eat and your glucose level is in the target range but you have two arrows going up, you might consider increasing your meal insulin dosage or increasing the time between your bolus and starting your meal. If you are going to take a correction dose, you might

consider increasing or decreasing per the arrows: 5% up or down for 1 arrow, or 10% up or down for 2 arrows. However, precaution should always be taken at night if you increase your dose of insulin.

Alarms and Alerts

Alarms and alerts add tremendous value, but they must be set correctly. If the alarms and alerts are not set correctly, you may have alarms going off all the time, which will make you eventually so used to hearing them that you don't pay attention to them or even notice them (this is called "alarm fatigue"). Moreover, your alarms and alerts will change from your initial settings as you gain more experience using a CGM. Alarms and alerts help with the early detection of glucose values heading out of the target range. They can warn you when you are about to go out of the target range (these are called "predictive alerts") or when glucose values are changing rapidly (these are called "rate-of-change alerts"). They are especially valuable if you have trouble recognizing low glucose levels ("hypoglycemia unawareness"), rapidly falling glucose levels, or concerns about hyperglycemia. Most alarms can be programmed, so you can set your high and low glucose thresholds, how early you want the predictive alarm to go off (generally 20 or 30 minutes before you reach a specified value), and if you want them to repeat.

All alarms take several button pushes or keystrokes to disable, ensuring that they are not accidentally turned off and that you notice the alarm. Alarms can be set to different volumes. Here are all of the alarms that are available for the CGM:

• Threshold alarm: high or low glucose level reached

• Predictive high and low alarms: about to go out of target range

• Rate-of-change alarm: levels are rising or falling rapidly

• Low-battery (receiver or transmitter) alarm: battery will need to be recharged or replaced

• Lost sensor alarm: the CGM has lost the signal from the sensor and transmitter

• Weak signal alarm: the CGM is not receiving a strong signal from the sensor and transmitter

More Details About Alarms

Low-Glucose Threshold Alarm. When you first begin using a CGM, you may want to only set the low-glucose threshold alarm. Provided you don't have hypoglycemia unawareness, you may want to set it at a relatively low value, until you get used to the CGM and its alarms. As you become more experienced, you will want to increase this threshold, so you can help keep your glucose levels under tighter control.

High-Glucose Threshold Alarm. You might not want to set a high-glucose threshold alarm when you first start using a CGM. As you gain experience and as your glucose levels improve, you may set this threshold rather high—around 300 mg/dL—and then gradually decrease it to help prevent high glucose levels. Eventually, you might set this alarm at the upper level for your target range to better manage your glucose levels.

Predictive High and Low Alarms. You should not set predictive high and low alarms at the beginning of CGM use. These alarms should be set once you have your threshold alarms at the levels that work best for you. Set the predictive alarm to notify you if you are going to reach your high or low threshold in 10 minutes (or 20–30 mg/dL [1.1–1.6 mmol/L] below your high glucose threshold so you are alerted to an impending hyperglycemic glucose level). Once you get used to this setting and succeed in using the CGM to prevent high and low levels, you might want to increase the time frame to 15 or 20 minutes, or 40–60 mg/dL (2.2–3.3 mmol/L). With predictive alarms, you have to get used to the fact that they might go off when your glucose level is still normal but on its way out of your target range. You can administer a small bolus to avert rising glucose levels or take a small amount of carbohydrate to prevent going low. After treating, view your trend graph and trend arrows to be sure that you are averting hitting the threshold. If not, the threshold alarm will sound.

Rate-of-Change Alarm. This is the last alarm you will set on the CGM. Wait until you are familiar with all of the other alarms and they are at their optimal settings. The rate-of-change alarm goes off when your glucose is trending up or down at a rapid rate. It may go off when your glucose level is in your target range. When rate-of-change alarms are used successfully, they can help you completely avoid highs and lows by giving you enough warning to treat your glucose when it is trending high (take a small correction bolus or temporarily increase your basal rate) or trending low (take extra carbohydrate or temporarily decrease your basal rate). The high rate-of-change alarm helps if you frequently miss meal boluses. This alarm will sound as your glucose is starting rise from your meal, allowing you to take the meal bolus—and even though it will be late, it will be better than no meal bolus at all.

Threshold-Suspend and Predictive-Suspend Alarms. In addition to giving alarms and alerts, a CGM can, in certain newer pumps, also tell the pump to stop basal insulin delivery at a preset or predicted low threshold. The first devices commercially available have a range for insulin suspension, a fixed maximal time period for suspension (2 hours), and the ability for the patient to intervene at any time and restart basal insulin. The present devices all have a fixed alarm if the preset threshold is reached. There is also a predictive suspend that stops basal insulin in anticipation of approaching the threshold with a predictive horizon of 30 minutes. This functionality can also turn basal insulin delivery back on automatically within 30–120 minutes if the glucose value recovers per a specific algorithm (mathematical equations). In addition, you can always turn basal insulin on and stop the suspend if you choose to treat your low or impending low glucose with glucose by mouth. Keep in mind these are integrated systems and only the one CGM that is part of the system works to suspend insulin automatically by the pump.

Hybrid Closed-Loop Alarms. One recently approved system has a CGM that will not only suspend insulin delivery, but also determine how the pump gives basal insulin per a control algorithm (mathematical equations). At the present time, there are multiple systems in development and only one approved for use commercially. These closed-loop systems that automate insulin delivery, mainly for basal insulin replacement, still require patients to bolus for their meals, calibrate their sensors, and respond to alarms for certain conditions, such as prolonged hypoglycemia or hyperglycemia, or sensor or system issues. For more about closed-loop systems, see Chapter 12.

Graphs

You can view graphs of your glucose levels (sensor glucose on the x-axis, horizontally, and time on the y-axis, vertically) on your CGM. Graphs display your sensor glucose levels over various time periods: 3, 6, 12, and 24 hours. The display indicates your target range, so you can see if the CGM readings are in target. CGMs have companion software that you can use to review several days' worth of information on your computer. The receiver stores the information, even though you cannot see it on the monitor itself. Learning how to review this information is essential to improving your glucose control. How to download and assess your CGM data is covered later.

Current Value

Your current sensor glucose value is displayed on the home or first screen that comes up when you activate the monitor. This information updates every 5 minutes.

WHAT'S INVOLVED WITH WEARING A CGM?

There are some daily maintenance tasks that you will need to do to ensure that your sensor is functioning properly and staying in place. As with an insulin pump, doing a quick assessment of your sensor every day will help prevent sudden problems and lower the odds of you having to do a lot of troubleshooting.

Inserting the Sensor

Begin by prepping your skin, loading the injector, and applying any topical adhesive aids. Insert the sensor, and cover the area with tape afterward. Be sure to be thorough with rubbing the tape once it is inserted. The heat and pressure from rubbing the tape helps it stick better. Put the transmitter in place, tell the receiver that you have inserted a new sensor, and wait for it to receive the signal from the new sensor. When it "finds" the new sensor, there is a warm-up period that will last 2 hours.

This warm-up period allows any swelling at the site of insertion to go down and decreases the chances that your first calibration results in error. After this warm-up period, the receiver will ask for a blood glucose calibration from self-monitoring of blood glucose (SMBG). For this calibration, you must test your blood glucose with a meter. The meter can be linked through radio frequency to the CGM receiver, or wholly separate. The CGM algorithms (formulas) calibrate the sensor according to the glucose reading from SMBG. This step determines the glucose value that shows up on the CGM receiver screen.

Each CGM device is slightly different, but most require calibration two times a day (or every 12 hours).

Each sensor and its associated injector have specific loading methods. Some injectors are spring-loaded; in others, you must insert the sensor manually via the inserter. After the sensor is inserted and the needle has been removed, check the site for bleeding. Some bleeding is normal. If there is bleeding, dab it with the corner of a tissue or cloth until it stops. Do not attach the transmitter to the sensor until the bleeding has stopped—not doing so could affect the accuracy of the device. Once the bleeding has stopped, attach the transmitter to the sensor. If the bleeding won't stop or it starts to leak out the top of the sensor platform, you may need to insert a new sensor. The transmitter can technically be worn by just

REMEMBER!

Your sensor, transmitter, and receiver are all technology and can be fragile! Treat them with care, and avoid putting them into places where they might get cracked or scratched (e.g., a purse or luggage) and try to avoid dropping them.

clipping it into the sensor, but it is highly recommended that you place more tape over the top. You don't want to lose the transmitter; it is expensive. Try different ways to secure it.

You might have to experiment a lot to find the best way to attach and secure your CGM. Make sure to read the instructions that come with your CGM, or reach out to your device trainer for help. For some brands, covering the whole transmitter with tape is not advised. See the section at the end of this chapter called "Tips for Taping and Keeping Your Sensor On" for more help.

Once your sensor is attached and has been secured and calibrated, it will send real-time CGM data, which can be seen on the receiver. While you are wearing the sensor, you need to check how it is functioning and how you are reacting to it at periodic intervals. Check to be sure that it is securely attached, that the batteries of the transmitter and receiver are charged and working, and that your skin is healthy (not red and no swelling and pain present). Remember, it is critical to calibrate the sensor with an SMBG reading when the sensor requests it. Once you obtain your SMBG reading, calibrate the CGM within 5 minutes. If you wait longer, the SMBG reading you just obtained may no longer be accurate as your glucose level fluctuates. Try to calibrate before you go to bed, so you can avoid waking up to a calibration alarm or a nonfunctioning sensor if you sleep through the alarm.

After 6 or 7 days, most sensors will expire. Remove the sensor and transmitter, recharge the transmitter batteries (if necessary), and take care of your skin—you will likely need that spot again soon. If your sensor or transmitter falls off or comes out, do not reuse that sensor. You cannot reinsert a used sensor. Once finished with your sensor, remove the transmitter and put the sensor part in your sharps disposal container.

Charging the transmitter at this time is a good idea. If the battery on your transmitter goes out in the middle of a sensor's life, it can end the sensor's life as well. It's smart to always check battery life before you insert a new sensor so that you don't waste one because of a dead or low-charged battery. Some CGM transmitters don't require recharging but use batteries that last for months.

Costs

The technology needed to run a CGM system with the three components is fairly advanced. The receiver is a one-time purchase (within warranty), the transmitters need to be replaced between one and four times per year, and the sensors only last 6–7 days. Therefore, it is important for you to determine what you will have to pay for a CGM and what you are willing to pay. Call your insurance company and ask to speak to someone who is familiar with your plan's policy on diabetes supplies. You must have a prescription for a CGM. Only you and your diabetes team can assess whether you (and your family) are ready for a CGM. You and your team should also be able to determine which device will work best for you. They should help set up your training—either by doing it themselves or with a representative from the CGM manufacturer. Training takes from 3 to 6 hours.

You should anticipate follow-up visits, calls, or e-mails to adjust alarms, to adjust your insulin regimen, and to discuss your treatment plan for high and low glucose levels. Uploading and reviewing the data will help you and your diabetes team examine and understand your glucose levels, what is associated with high and low levels, and strategies to improve your diabetes management. Getting a CGM can improve diabetes control in people with type 1 diabetes when it is properly used and the data are effectively reviewed. By adjusting your diabetes regimen in response to your glucose trends and patterns—and by using real-time values and alerts and alarms—you can make your journey with diabetes the best and safest that it possibly can be.

TIPS FOR TAPING AND KEEPING YOUR SENSOR ON

CGM sensors and transmitters are expensive, and they are valuable for glucose management. In some instances, receivers are designed to last around 1 year, and it may be that long before insurance will replace a lost or nonfunctioning device. Therefore, it is imperative to keep the sensor platform and transmitter well adhered to the skin so that they are not lost! There are a few tricks that people have

IMPORTANT TIPS THAT CAN AFFECT THE ADHERENCE OF THE SENSOR TAPE

- Keep the skin clean and dry, free from lotions, soaps, and oils.
- Think about the amount of hair you have at the sensor location (shave it down before insertion if hair impedes sticking).
- If you are a person who sweats a lot, you may want to apply antiperspirant to the area.
- Apply pressure and rub the tape once inserted.
- Use more tape!

developed to help keep sensors in place, and companies are coming out with new patches specifically designed to help keep sensors locked into place.

The sensor platform comes with its own small piece of tape. For some, this is the only tape needed for the sensor to remain in place for the expected amount of time; others seem to need more tape to keep it on. This sensor platform tape is designed to be activated by heat and pressure. This means that when you insert and *before* you put on the transmitter, rub the tape with firm, even pressure for about 15–30 seconds over the whole area. This step will help your sensor stick right off the bat. If you need further assistance keeping your sensor on, the following information may help you.

Do not apply oils, lotions, or creamy soaps in the area and on the day you plan on inserting a new sensor. The best time to insert is after a shower or bath so that the skin is clean, but make sure you wait about 30 minutes after a shower before inserting a new CGM. Waiting 30 minutes will ensure your skin is dry. Also, use an alcohol wipe in the area of insertion to clean off any residue just before insertion (let this dry, too). Wait at least 30–45 minutes after inserting to take a shower as well. The tape hasn't had the appropriate time to adhere yet, and it will fall off.

Some people like to use tape underneath or use other solvent adhesive aids like barrier films (these are products that can be used for pump sites, too). These products generally come in a swab or wipe and are applied like alcohol. Insert the sensor while these barrier films are still slightly tacky/wet for the best adherence (and again remember to rub the sensor tape). You may also want to try a piece of stronger tape under the sensor's tape if you know that type of adhesive works better on your skin. The most important thing to remember if you use barrier film or another adhesive under the sensor is that you cannot insert through it. If you are using barrier film, draw a small circle on your skin where you plan to insert, and apply a barrier around it. With tape, cut a small hole in it before placing it on your skin and insert the sensor through that. If you insert through other tapes, it may damage the sensor and create false glucose readings, resulting in trashing your sensor early.

If you are inserting the sensor in a place that has a lot of hair, consider shaving or trimming down the hair (or even wax it!). If you perspire a lot, an unscented spray or solid antiperspirant might help. For this option, use the product on your skin several hours before sensor insertion, and then be sure to thoroughly clean the area before placing the sensor.

For tape that covers the CGM once inserted, you can use a "window" technique. Cut four strips of tape and place them one-by-one around the transmitter, in the shape of a window, making sure to cover the original tape on the CGM platform but not the transmitter itself. Another option is to cut a hole the size of your transmitter in the tape piece and place it so that it doesn't cover the transmitter completely.

There are several companies that make transparent dressings for intravenous sites for hospitals. These dressings are made to stick to skin, allow for visualization through to the device (they are transparent), and stretch and move with skin and are designed to be removed without much pain. For these products, remove them by pulling out/away from the center on the tape, rather than up. This stretches the dressing and releases the hold it had.

Other options are sports tapes or bands that would hold the sensor and transmitter in place. There are companies who custom cut tape in various shapes and colors designed to fit over sensors and various pump sites. They tend to cater to young kids but have a wide variety of options. A quick look through the diabetes blogosphere for ideas regarding keeping CGMs on will yield good results.

For activities like swimming or surfing, double-check your tape's integrity before going out. If your CGM is on your arm, you may need to wrap a sweatband, co-band, more tape, or another wrap around your CGM to help keep it in place even if the adhesive starts to loosen.

For skin reactions to the tape or the sensor, using a tape on the skin first may decrease skin exposure to irritants. The use of a steroid spray, such as that used for nasal allergies, might also be of benefit, especially if the reaction is red and itchy.

CHAPTER REVIEW

➡ A CGM generates a lot of data. There are trend arrows, alarms, alerts, graphs, and the current sensor glucose value. Using CGM data effectively will allow you to get the best results out of your CGM and your diabetes management.

➡ There are some maintenance tasks you need to do daily to ensure that your sensor is functioning properly and staying in place. As with an insulin pump, do a quick assessment of your sensor every day to help prevent problems and reduce the amount of potential troubleshooting. You also need to know how to properly insert your sensor and ensure that it stays on.

➡ Using a CGM can improve your diabetes control when properly used and understood. By adjusting your diabetes regimen in response to the glucose trends and patterns provided by a CGM, and by taking advantage of real-time values and alerts and alarms, you can make your journey with diabetes the best and safest that it can be.

➡ Tips on how to keep your sensor taped on securely include removing oils or lotions, making sure your skin is dry and clean, and, if needed, trying the many different barriers, extra tapes, and glue-like wipes to see what works best.

➡ If you use CGM intermittently, be careful when you are without it. It is likely that you have become dependent on the continuous glucose display, the trend arrows, and the alarms—and without them, you put yourself at risk for fluctuations in glucose levels and even severe hypoglycemia, or diabetic ketoacidosis (DKA).

CASE STUDY: USING CONTINUOUS GLUCOSE MONITORING FOR OVERNIGHT BASAL RATE CHANGES

JOSH

Josh started waking up in the mornings with low glucose levels. He talked to his health care providers, and they agreed to use a retrospective or diagnostic CGM to better characterize his hypoglycemia. When his data were uploaded, they showed that his glucose fell below 70 mg/dL between 12:00 A.M. and 3:00 A.M. on Monday, Wednesday, and Friday and often stayed that low until he woke up at 6:00 A.M. He also noticed that his overnight glucose levels on Tuesday, Thursday, and the weekend did not have a low pattern. Josh wasn't surprised, since he routinely went to the gym after work on Monday, Wednesday, and Friday.

Josh and his doctor decided to decrease his insulin pump basal rates on the nights he exercised. They set up a new pattern on his insulin pump, decreasing his basal rates by 15% (85% of his normal amount would still be given) for 3 hours, starting 1 hour before the gym and ending 1 hour after his workout. They also decreased his nighttime basal rate by 20% from 10:00 P.M. (2 hours before he started going low) to 4:00 A.M. (2 hours before he woke up). Josh set a Monday, Wednesday, and Friday late-afternoon reminder on his phone to change to his new basal pattern.

They decided Josh would start to use a real-time CGM with a predictive alarm set at 70 mg/dL at 30 minutes. Josh felt this would give him ample time to take some carbohydrate and protein to avert hypoglycemia. The first time wearing the real-time sensor, Josh's predictive low alert went off within 1–2 hours of starting exercise. This alert prompted Josh to decrease his basal rate during exercise by 20% (instead of 15%). Josh also noticed that on Tuesday and Thursday mornings, he woke up with a high glucose level, which started to climb around the 3:00 A.M. time frame.

Josh decreased the time frame for his reduced basal rate to 1:00 A.M. (2 hours before his glucose started to increase) and also changed the nighttime basal rate from a 20% decrease to a 15% reduction. Josh also decided to set a high alert starting at 2:00 A.M. at 250 mg/dL, so he could treat an early morning high glucose if needed.

IN THIS CHAPTER

CHAPTER 12

HYBRID CLOSED-LOOP SYSTEMS

Early research suggests that closed-loop technology may improve diabetes outcomes: there is more time in-target for glucose levels, with less time in the hypoglycemic and hyperglycemic ranges. While there are only a few studies of long enough duration to assess A1C, the findings suggest that A1C values improve in some users with the automation of insulin delivery. In addition, they decrease the burden of diabetes management for patients.

INTRODUCING THE CONCEPT OF HYBRID CLOSED-LOOP SYSTEMS

Hybrid closed-loop systems are a new type of diabetes treatment that use technology to deliver basal insulin in a different way than traditional insulin pumps (traditional pumps are open-loop). These closed-loop systems automate the delivery of insulin through control algorithms (mathematical formulas). The algorithms take into account the sensor glucose data—what the glucose level is now, the rate of change of the glucose value, and where the glucose level is predicted to be—to determine how much insulin to deliver every 5 minutes. The algorithms also account for how much insulin is on board and insulin sensitivity. This basal insulin delivery is different than the preprogrammed basal rate insulin delivery in the open-loop. In addition, the control algorithms target a specific glucose level or range. The first commercially available system targets getting the glucose level to 120 mg/dL in its mathematical calculations. The device also has a temporary target of 150 mg/dL that can be set

> When the system is using a control algorithm to determine insulin delivery, it is termed to be in "closed-loop" or "auto mode."

for exercise, or other conditions in which hypoglycemia might be a heightened risk, such as during illness or while traveling.

COMPONENTS OF HYBRID CLOSED-LOOP SYSTEMS

Closed-loop systems have three main components: an insulin pump, a continuous glucose monitor (CGM), and a control algorithm (mathematical formula). The algorithm uses information from the CGM and the pump to dictate basal insulin delivery. The algorithm may be housed in the insulin pump or in a separate handheld device. The goals of closed-loop systems are to reduce the burden of diabetes management and to improve diabetes outcomes for people.

HOW HYBRID CLOSED-LOOP SYSTEMS WORK

The first system that is available is called a hybrid closed-loop system. It is called a "hybrid" system because users still need to count carbohydrates, deliver meal and snack insulin (optimally before starting to eat), and confirm correction doses for high glucose levels; the system does not control all insulin dosing. Many groups are working to develop fully closed-loop systems that will automatically deliver meal insulin and require little from the patient with regard to diabetes management. However, one of the major barriers to developing such fully closed-loop systems is the slow absorption of insulin from the subcutaneous space.

The Algorithm

There is one hybrid closed-loop system that has been approved for commercial use at the writing of this second edition, although several others are expected to come to market in the near future.

It uses an algorithm that replaces basal rates with microbasal dosing that occurs every 5 minutes. Each 5-minute microbasal dose can be a different amount that doesn't usually add up to the preset hourly basal rates of an open-loop. These individual microbasal doses can be as low as zero and as high as a level determined by the algorithm. There is a maximal amount of basal the system can deliver with each dose called the maximal automatic basal insulin delivery, or Umax. The calculation of each microbasal is based on several factors:

- The present sensor glucose level

- The sensor glucose rate of change

- Predicted sensor glucose levels

- How much total insulin was given in the past few hours (insulin on board)

- Recent total daily doses of insulin

- Glucose target(s)

- If the user has indicated he or she may be exercising and has put on a temporary target of 150 mg/dL

When a system does not have an accurate CGM value, the patient has been out of glycemic target too long, or if other safety criteria are not met, the algorithm turns off and the patient resumes his or her previously preprogrammed basal rates. When out of the closed-loop mode, the system will act as any other conventional pump. It will deliver preprogrammed basal rates (such as the ones you and your health care provider have already determined), and the CGM value has no effect on insulin administration.

The algorithm can give extra insulin as microboluses when sensor glucose values are high or predicted to be high and can suspend or decrease insulin when sensor glucose values are low or predicted to be low.

Rising Glucose Levels

When the algorithm predicts that the sensor glucose level will continue to rise and the insulin-on-board is not sufficient to bring it back into range, the microbasal amount is increased. Generally, there are safety measures for how much total insulin the microbasal can give in a certain time period, such as every 5 minutes for the one commercially available system. If the system cannot bring glucose levels back into range this way, a correction bolus can be given by the user that is derived by the algorithm. If high glucose levels are prolonged or if maximal insulin delivery occurs for too long a time, the closed-loop mode may be suspended. You can then clear the alarm and enter a fingerstick glucose level; the pump can resume closed-loop mode again.

Dropping Glucose Levels

If glucose levels are dropping or are low, the algorithm can suspend microbasal insulin; however, there is a maximal amount of time for suspension, which differs depending on the closed-loop system. Suspending insulin has been shown to greatly reduce hypoglycemia, especially at night.

THE IMPORTANCE OF THE CGM

Hybrid closed-loop systems use sensor glucose information to make basal dosing adjustments. The accuracy and reliability of the CGM value is paramount for closed-loop mode to operate correctly. If CGM readings are inconsistent, the CGM value is off from what the most recent calibration value was, or if it meets any other predetermined safety criteria, the system will exit closed-loop. So keeping your CGM calibrated, and correctly taped, will better ensure that you remain in the closed-loop mode as much as possible.

Hybrid closed-loop systems are examples of making insulin dosing decisions based off of CGM values. We've come a long way in terms of CGM accuracy and capabilities!

When you first start hybrid closed-loop mode, some systems require time on the pump in open-loop first to gather data on your insulin delivery. This step could be as short as 2 days. Other systems may be able to transition from open- to closed-loop by knowing your weight. During the first days of hybrid closed-loop, the system is familiarizing itself with your glucose trends and patterns and how much insulin you require—in other words, adapting to you. Therefore, the first few days might not be as optimal as hybrid closed-loop becomes over time.

CHAPTER REVIEW

➡ If you wear your sensor consistently and keep it taped and calibrated, you could remain in hybrid closed-loop mode nearly all of the time.

➡ There could be times when you are not in hybrid closed-loop mode because of device issues with the pump, the sensor, or transmitter.

➡ If you are suddenly in a situation where hybrid closed-loop mode is not available, you will need accurate basal rates to fall back on. Try to remember to reassess your basal rates periodically when you use a hybrid closed-loop system.

➡ Hybrid closed-loop technology is an advancement in diabetes therapy, and studies to date have shown that glucose levels improve with more time in-target, and there is less hypoglycemia and hyperglycemia.

SECTION 4:
ILLNESS, TRAVEL, AND SCHOOL

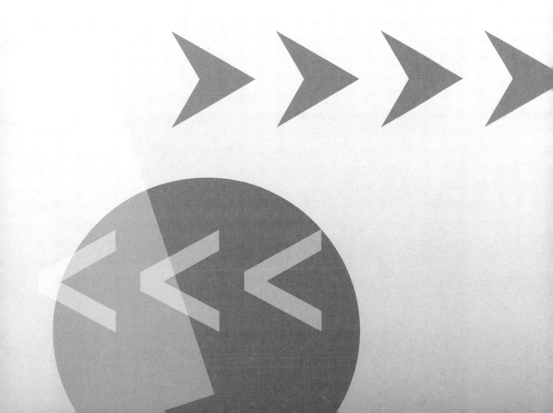

IN THIS CHAPTER

➡ Sick Days

➡ Troubleshooting High and Low Glucose Levels

➡ Hyperglycemia and Ketones

➡ Hospital Visits

➡ Time Off the Pump or CGM

CHAPTER 13

SPECIAL CIRCUMSTANCES: SICK DAYS, IN-HOSPITAL USE, AND DISCONTINUING PUMP THERAPY

Paying attention to your diabetes when you're sick or in need of hospitalization is always important. It is no less important when you're on insulin pump therapy. In fact, in many ways, it may be easier. With an insulin pump and meticulous glucose monitoring or the use of a continuous glucose monitor (CGM), you can quickly make changes in insulin delivery to avoid episodes of hypoglycemia and hyperglycemia that could complicate your illness or delay your recovery.

SICK DAYS

When you have diabetes, an illness can make your glucose control difficult. When your body is stressed by illness, particularly when you are vomiting, have diarrhea, or have a fever, your body releases hormones (counterregulatory hormones) that order your liver to release stored glucose and tell your fat to release free fatty acids to form ketones. Your body does this when you're sick because you need more energy to fight off infection and to repair damaged tissue. If you don't have diabetes, your body releases more insulin to control the rise in glucose and ketones. When you have diabetes, you need to manage the process on your own, by monitoring your glucose and ketone levels and by increasing insulin delivery to manage the situation. In addition, you are at risk of hypoglycemia when you are ill, particularly if you don't eat or drink, are vomiting, or have diarrhea. Either way, if you don't control glucose and ketones, you can end up developing diabetic ketoacidosis (DKA), or severe

CATEGORIES OF ILLNESS

Illnesses are broken down into two categories:

1. Illnesses that can potentially lead to dehydration and are accompanied by lack of appetite, nausea, vomiting, or diarrhea
2. Illnesses that don't increase the risk of dehydration, such as colds

hypoglycemia. DKA can make you much sicker, potentially requiring a prolonged hospitalization, and delay your recovery.

Illnesses with Risk of Dehydration

Dehydrating illnesses can be more dangerous if you have diabetes. They require more attention and possibly a call or visit to your health care team. This group includes illnesses that lead to reduced intake of fluids (fluids are more important than food), nausea, vomiting, or diarrhea. If your blood glucose is going low or is already low because of such an illness, temporarily reduce your basal rate by 25–50%. If you need to suspend insulin delivery, don't suspend it for more than 30 minutes or you will increase the risk of developing ketones. If hypoglycemia continues, you might consider administering a low dose of glucagon, but before you do this, you will need to discuss this approach with your health care team.

If your glucose level is high, you must maintain a balance between increasing insulin delivery and maintaining hydration, remembering that if your glucose level is above 180–200 mg/dL, then you will likely urinate more often because of the glucose being excreted in your urine. A temporary basal rate with a 25–50% increase or a small correction bolus (but less than what is calculated by the pump's bolus calculator) may be enough to bring your blood glucose level back down into your target range. However, you don't want to bring your glucose level down too low because you could develop hypoglycemia. Developing hypoglycemia is especially a problem if you are unable to keep down fluids, which would make it difficult to treat low glucose.

LOW-DOSE OR MINI-DOSE GLUCAGON
Dose:
- 2 units (20 mg) for children aged 2 years or younger
- 1 unit (10 mg) per year of age for children aged 3–15 years
- 15 units (150 mg) for children older than 15 years

Raises the glucose level 50–200 mg/dL in around 30 minutes.

Dosing is done by age and measured in units on the insulin syringe; 1 unit equals 10 mg glucagon.

Illnesses That Don't Increase Risk of Dehydration
This category of illnesses is less worrisome, and the goal is to get your glucose level to just below the upper range of your target, avoiding both hyperglycemia and hypoglycemia. Continue to drink to stay hydrated when you are ill.

Sick-Day Treatments
The basic treatments for sick days on the pump are similar to what you did before on multiple daily injections (MDI). Below are some key things to keep in mind.

Start a Log
Keep track of the following:
- Glucose levels
- Ketones
- Temperature
- Oral intake of fluids with carbohydrate/glucose count grams of carbohydrate/glucose ingested)
- Oral intake of fluids without carbohydrate/glucose (fluids are important for maintaining hydration)
- Urination
- Episodes of vomiting or diarrhea
- Any medication taken, amount, and time

Check Your Glucose Level Often

Monitor your glucose levels very closely, every 1–2 hours. You might need to check every 30 minutes if your glucose levels are changing rapidly. If you are using a CGM, look at the trend and absolute value every 10–15 minutes. The goal is to keep your glucose at the upper level of your target range and to avoid hypoglycemia and hyperglycemia.

Stay Hydrated by Drinking Fluids

It's easy to become dehydrated when you're sick. Dehydration results from vomiting, diarrhea, and hyperglycemia. If your glucose level is above 180–200 mg/dL, you will urinate more often as your body tries to flush out the extra glucose through your urine. After vomiting, wait 30–60 minutes, and then start hydrating yourself with teaspoons of water or ice chips, progressing to tablespoons, and then to ounces. When your glucose level is below 150 mg/dL, treat it with glucose-containing fluids, such as sports drinks, electrolyte-containing liquids, or flat sugar-containing sodas without caffeine. The goal is to try to retain 4–6 oz of fluids (2–4 oz for younger children) every 30–60 minutes until you are rehydrated.

Continue to Take Your Insulin

This is very important. Your body still needs insulin to use the sugar in your blood for energy, and you need all the energy you can get when you are sick. Even if you are not eating or drinking fluids with carbohydrate, you still need insulin. You might even need more insulin because the stress hormones released in response to illness can cause blood glucose levels to increase.

Check Ketones at the Beginning of and Periodically During Your Illness

When you're sick, your body may start to break down fat for energy. When this happens, ketones are produced. Ketones may develop even if your glucose level isn't high. If ketones are present, check every time you urinate, or every 4 hours if you are monitoring ketones in blood. If ketones are not present, check for them two times a day until you are well. If you become nauseated or begin vomiting, check again; these can be signs of the presence of ketones. It is very important to know if ketones are present because this means you need more fluid, more insulin, and more glucose if your blood glucose level is below 150–200 mg/dL.

Check Your Pump Site and Tubing

Changing your set when you become sick is a good idea so you know that your site is working, your site absorption is adequate, and your cannula is not kinked or bent. By starting out with a fresh site, you have a better chance of having your insulin absorbed correctly when you need it most. If you just changed your set, look for bubbles and maybe add some extra tape for security. If glucose values are not coming down and your infusion set seems to be working, for peace of mind and to know you are receiving all the insulin you intend to, you may want to switch to insulin injections. Just remember to log the time and amount of insulin given via shot.

Let Others Know What to Do When You Are Ill

If you become too sick to check your glucose and manage your diabetes, you need help.

Help can come in three ways:

1. Someone who has been taught (your spouse, best friend, roommate, parents, etc.) how to check your glucose, deliver insulin via your pump, administer glucagon, and more. In other words, someone else knows how to manage your diabetes, and they are prepared to help you while you are ill.

2. Someone who knows how to check and interpret your glucose levels, how to give you glucose orally, and when to call for help.

3. Someone who knows how to call for help, either from your diabetes team or 911.

The more people who can help you manage your diabetes, the safer you will be during an illness or accident.

A GOOD IDEA

It is a good idea to teach someone how to disconnect or suspend your pump if you develop severe hypoglycemia and are unable to treat yourself. But this person must also know that you might need glucagon or emergency services by calling 911.

Your Glucose Level and Some Medications

Some medications, such as inhalers for asthma or steroid-based pain medications, might increase your glucose level. Before taking medications, discuss the effect the medication might have on your diabetes management with your health care team. If a certain medication is known to increase glucose levels, discuss whether you should increase your basal rates or just rely on correction doses. Some medications also contain sugar for flavoring. Sugared cough drops can have up to 5 grams of carbohydrate per lozenge! Take the necessary amount of insulin for these types of medications, and as always, test often and record what you find.

TROUBLESHOOTING HIGH AND LOW GLUCOSE LEVELS

You should develop a routine to troubleshoot high glucose levels. This routine should include checking your infusion site, the infusion set tubing, the connection between your reservoir and infusion set, the reservoir itself, the effectiveness of your insulin (is it expired or has it been exposed to excessive cold or heat?), and the insulin pump. The table on page 185 lists what to check, what questions to ask yourself, and what to do.

In addition, you should assess your own health and well-being. Ask yourself if you feel like you are getting sick. Did you take any medications? Are you stressed? If you are a menstruating woman, are you about to get your period? If something is going on with your overall health status, you may want to contact your diabetes team or prepare for sick-day management.

Troubleshooting Guidelines

What to Check	Questions to Ask	If Yes...
Infusion site	– Is it red, irritated, or painful? – Is it wet or does it smell like insulin?	Change infusion set, reservoir, and insulin.
Infusion set tubing	– Are there bubbles (larger than champagne bubbles) in the tubing? – Is there blood in the tubing?	Change infusion set, reservoir, and insulin.
Connection between reservoir and infusion set	– Are there leaks or breaks? – Is connection loose or easily moved?	Change infusion set, reservoir, and insulin if unable to correct the problem by tightening.
Reservoir or cartridge	– Is it loaded correctly? – Is the reservoir empty? – Are there excessive bubbles?	Change infusion set, reservoir, and insulin if unable to correct the issue.
Insulin	– Has insulin vial expired? – Has insulin been exposed to high temperatures or direct sunlight for longer than 30 minutes?	Change infusion set and reservoir, using a new vial of insulin. (When in doubt, change it out!)
Check insulin pump settings – Bolus delivery – Basal rates – Time	– Was last meal bolus missed? – Are basal rates set incorrectly? – Is time set incorrectly?	– Give correction dose – Reset basal rates – Set time correctly
Insulin pump	– Is insulin pump not working or inoperable? – Not sure if insulin pump has a problem?	Call the toll-free help line for your insulin pump manufacturer. The number is often located on the pump itself.

You can also help your troubleshooting along if you know what can cause hypoglycemia (low blood glucose) and hyperglycemia (high blood glucose) when you use an insulin pump.

HYPERGLYCEMIA AND KETONES

Whenever glucose levels are above 250 mg/dL, you should check for ketones. Whether the test for ketones is positive or negative will determine how you should treat the elevated blood glucose.

Ketones are acids made up of acetoacetic acid and β-hydroxybutyric acid and are sometimes called ketoacids. They are made when fat is broken down. Fatty acids are freed from fat, and then the liver makes them into ketones. The body forms these ketones when it is trying to produce more fuel because there isn't enough energy being received from metabolized glucose and glycogen (glucose stores released from the liver). When ketones build up in your bloodstream, you have ketosis and are at risk of developing DKA, a serious and potentially life-threatening condition.

You develop ketones when you do not have enough insulin in your bloodstream. You can develop ketones, even if you take your usual dose of insulin, if the amount you took does not meet your metabolic

Causes of Hypoglycemia and Hyperglycemia While on an Insulin Pump

Hyperglycemia	Hypoglycemia
Too little insulin given as bolus	Too much insulin given as boluses
• Incorrect CR for corrections	• Incorrect CR for corrections
• Incorrect CR for food	• Incorrect CR for food
• Underestimating food intake	• Overestimating food intake
• Missed bolus	• Insulin stacking
• Manual bolusing	• Manual bolusing
• Delayed timing of food bolus	• Delayed eating after bolus
Basal rates have not been increased as needed	Basal rates are too high
• Basal infusion rates too low	• Need different pattern
• Need temporary increase or different pattern	• Need temporary decrease
Infusion set problems	Infusion set problems
• Cannula kinked or dislodged	• Not disconnected from body when priming or filling tubing
• Poor site with inadequate absorption	
• Inflammation or infection at the site	
• Air bubbles	
Other causes	Other causes
• Insulin expired or spoiled from heating or freezing	• Pump clock is wrong
• Pump malfunction	• Primed while attached
• Battery failure	

CR, carbohydrate ratio

needs at the time. Ketones develop with infection, stress, or illness. Commonly, the body makes ketones when glucose levels are very high. However, you may have only mildly elevated glucose, a normal glucose level, or even a low glucose value (during starvation) and still produce ketones. Your body tries to eliminate ketones through breathing (your breathing becomes deep and labored and the ketones make your breath smell like rotting fruit) and urination (causing you also to lose important electrolytes, like potassium and sodium).

It is important for everyone using insulin pump therapy to understand that they can develop ketones if the pump stops delivering insulin. This is because there will no longer be any long-acting or basal insulin in the body. Ketones may form as quickly as 3 hours after insulin interruption. If you have an infusion-set malfunction or blocked tubing or cannula, you may not realize that you are not receiving insulin. You may know only when you find a high glucose level and then check for ketones.

When blood glucose is ≥250 mg/dL, check for KETONES and follow these guidelines.

Positive for ketones (or if nauseated, vomiting, urinating excessively, or have fruity-smelling breath)	Negative for ketones

• Give a correction dose by injection
• Change infusion set, reservoir, and insulin
• Check blood glucose every 1–2 hours and give insulin by injection until blood glucose levels are within target range
• If the glucose level is not going down and you have moderate to high ketones, nausea, vomiting, or difficulty breathing, call your health care provider or go to the emergency room
	• Give a correction dose through the insulin pump
	• Recheck blood glucose in 1 hour
	• If blood glucose has not decreased in 1 hour
	  – give an insulin injection
	  – change infusion set, reservoir, and insulin
	• Continue to check your blood glucose until glucose levels are within the desired range

In this situation, it is best to give insulin by syringe, in case the high glucose level is caused by an issue with the pump or any of its parts.	*The most common causes of unexplained hyperglycemia that does not respond to a correction bolus include a kinked or displaced cannula, an infusion set or reservoir issue, or a "bad" vial of insulin.*

Urine ketones can be detected with ketone strips. A small detection patch changes color according to the level of ketones present (negative, small, moderate, large, and very large). Blood ketones can be checked with a normal fingerstick by a special machine. Readings are in millimoles per liter (mmol/L) and range from 0.0 to ≥3.0. Checking blood ketones is more accurate and a better way to quantify the levels of ketones.

With ketones, extra insulin is given every 2–4 hours until you no longer have ketones. Insulin resistance can occur when you have ketosis (meaning that the insulin you take may be less effective), so extra insulin beyond your usual correction for high glucose may be needed. You should discuss this with your health care team, but here are some basic concepts:

Small to moderate ketones. Calculate your correction bolus for your glucose level. Add 5–10% of your total daily insulin (you can find this in the history or utilities/daily totals section of your pump). If this is your first high glucose with ketones, you can take this bolus by pump. Recheck after 1–2 hours. If this is your second high glucose with ketones, take the correction and additional insulin by syringe. Then change your set, make sure your reservoir is filled, and verify that your pump is working. Recheck in 1–2 hours. If improving, continue rechecking and taking correction insulin every 2–4 hours until you are negative for ketones. But you do need to keep in mind the effects of active insulin.

Large ketones. You should take your calculated insulin dose plus 10–20% of your daily insulin total by syringe. Change your set. Be sure that your reservoir is filled and your pump is working. Call your health care team and recheck both glucose and ketones after 1–2 hours.

KETONES AND HYPOGLYCEMIA

If ketones form and you have normal or low glucose, drink fluids that contain glucose. Don't take bolus insulin until your glucose level is high enough to require correction.

BLOOD KETONE MEASUREMENTS

- <0.6 mmol/L, normal
- 0.6–1.5 mmol/L, consider this indicative of impending DKA
- >1.5 mmol/L, likely DKA

DRINK FLUIDS! The more fluids you can drink, the easier it is to help your body flush out the ketones. Drink plenty of water or glucose-free liquids when your glucose is above 180–200 mg/dL. When your glucose level falls below 180 mg/dL, if you still have ketones, start drinking glucose-containing liquids. Juice, tea with sugar or honey, flat sugar-containing sodas, or frozen pops with sugar will all work. Take insulin to cover the glucose you are ingesting.

HOSPITAL VISITS

Elective Admission

If you are scheduled to go to the hospital for an elective admission, you need to discuss your insulin delivery plan ahead of time with your diabetes team and the team that will care for you in the hospital. Find out if the hospital will allow you to stay on your pump. If you decide to remain on your insulin pump, bring extra supplies—infusion sets (and inserters), reservoirs, batteries—to last you through the number of days you will be in the hospital. Write down or copy the download of all your pump settings. During your hospitalization, you might need to increase or decrease basal rates and boluses depending on your ability to eat and move about and the level of stress or illness. Be sure the infusion set is not located in a place where you will lie on it constantly, and be sure to check the site frequently for infection or irritation. If the hospital staff uses their own blood testing equipment, then ask for the results or consider also checking on your own blood glucose meter.

Emergency Room Visits and Emergency Hospitalizations

It is critical that you have a medical ID bracelet or necklace that tells people you have diabetes. The health care personnel you encounter in the emergency room and hospital must pay close attention to your glucose levels. The hospital staff must manage your diabetes, and one option is to continue on your insulin pump. Staff can retrieve your basal insulin infusion rates as well as your bolus history from your insulin pump. They can also find a history of your glucose levels in the pump or meter. These pieces of information will be helpful as providers develop your diabetes treatment plan and as they consult your diabetes team.

Surgery

Insulin pumps may be used during minor procedures but are usually not used during major surgery, particularly if there is going to be prolonged general anesthesia. You and/or a family member need to discuss your glucose monitoring and insulin delivery plans with your medical teams. You want to be sure that your glucose levels are checked often (at least every hour) before, during, and after the procedure. The physicians responsible for your diabetes management should know your insulin pump settings, since these settings should help inform them of how to manage your diabetes while you are off the pump and receiving insulin by injection or by vein. Depending on your surgery, you might also want to remove your infusion set. As soon as you are able, ask about how much insulin you have and are presently receiving and about your glucose control. As much as possible, participate in your diabetes care, or have someone else designated as your diabetes caretaker. You will be on medications that might alter your judgment after surgery. If you remove your pump for the surgery, talk to your nursing staff about where to keep it. The pump may be brought to the operating room with you, or it may need to be left in your room. If left in your room, ask if there is a safe or locked area you can use.

Pregnancy

Insulin pump therapy is an option during pregnancy and may be considered in the preconception period, when the goal is to intensify management, lower A1C, reduce hypoglycemia, and stabilize glucose levels to help create the best outcomes for the mother and the baby. A CGM may also be a useful tool to help pregnant women keep a close eye on glucose levels.

Insulin requirements change during pregnancy. In the first half of pregnancy, risk of hypoglycemia is greater than before pregnancy. In the last trimester, insulin resistance increases so that basal rates may need to be increased by 0.3–0.6 units per hour and the carbohydrate ratio may need to be increased by 50–100%. Target glucose and A1C levels may be lower during pregnancy, since high blood glucose levels can be harmful to the fetus. Pregnant women are also at greater risk for ketone buildup and, consequently, DKA. Therefore, troubleshooting highs is essential (a CGM may be helpful in detecting impending hyperglycemia). Site selection during pregnancy can be difficult, so careful attention should be paid to the skin, particularly if infusion sets are placed in the abdomen. CGM alarms may help reduce the time spent in the high or low glucose ranges.

Insulin pumps may be used during labor and delivery, but an infusion of insulin by vein may be required if hyperglycemia cannot be controlled. During active labor, insulin needs are often extremely low. After delivery, most women will resume their prepregnancy insulin doses, since the insulin resistance of late pregnancy has resolved.

Women should be encouraged to breast-feed. During nursing, basal rate reduction is usually required. A CGM will inform the nursing mother of the changes in her glucose levels as they occur so that she can take extra glucose as needed. The ability of women with type 1 diabetes to now have healthy pregnancies and babies is due to careful, attentive management of diabetes before and during pregnancy.

TIME OFF THE PUMP OR CGM

There are times when you just can't wear the pump (e.g., long days of water activity) or when you decide you want a break from the pump. Those types of days when you are disconnected for only a short period of time (less than 2 hours) are easily regulated with periodic boluses from the pump. If you are planning on a full day off the pump or you tend to have several days off the pump, you might want to consider some of the following options.

- **Partial pump vacation (disconnecting multiple times in a day).** If you want to leave the infusion set in but only use the pump intermittently, you can take some basal insulin by injection to help reduce the risk of extreme high or low levels while you are disconnected. For example, taking a few units of basal insulin by injection will help keep glucose levels down during all-day sporting events or days at the beach. You must remember to reconnect and take supplemental insulin because these few units won't replace your full basal dose. You should also make sure that you reduce your total basal rate to compensate for the insulin you already have in your system from the injected insulin.

- **Total pump vacation.** If you want to completely remove your pump, you're going to have to return to MDI therapy. Talk to your health care team before you go back to MDI. To determine your dose of basal insulin by injection, you might want to take your total basal insulin used in the pump and increase it by 10–20%. Your boluses, which you will take by syringe, will be the same as what you took with your pump. If there are different carbohydrate ratios or correction factors used during different time periods, don't forget to follow those patterns. Be very careful not to stack insulin now that you don't have your bolus calculator (which uses active insulin to adjust correction boluses). Or get an app or a glucose meter that allows bolus calculations to be done.

- **Emergency discontinuation of insulin pump therapy.** If your pump stops working and it will take a day or two to get a replacement pump, you can manage your diabetes with MDI (go back to basal insulin once or twice a day and boluses for meals and correction) or with rapid-acting insulin only. If you choose to use rapid-acting insulin only, calculate and take your meal and correction boluses the same way you would if you were still on your pump. For your basal rate, you can calculate your basal insulin every 2 or

3 hours and take it as an injection at those time intervals. For example, if you had a basal rate of 1.1 units per hour from 6:00 to 9:00 A.M., you would take 3.3 units.

If you decide to take a break from the pump (regardless of which replacement method you're using), be sure that you always have insulin in your system. Insufficient insulin levels can lead to hyperglycemia and the development of ketones. Talk to your health care team if you want to take an extended vacation from the pump or if you decide the pump is not for you. They will help you return to the best diabetes management therapy for you.

PUMP DISCONNECTION GUIDELINES

1. Monitor glucose every 2 hours by SMBG or with CGM.
2. Consider taking a bolus equal to the basal insulin being missed (calculated as your basal rate multiplied by the number of hours you are off the pump) every 2–3 hours.
3. Reconnect for meals and corrections or take insulin by syringe.

CHAPTER REVIEW

➡ Sick-day management is critical when you are on an insulin pump. Be sure you have a protocol to follow and all the supplies you need, including a way to check ketones in blood or in urine. Start a log sheet, check glucose often (every 30–60 minutes initially), stay hydrated (drinking fluids matters more than eating), check ketones, check pump site and tubing, and be sure you have help. Contact your diabetes team as soon as is needed.

➡ If you have unexplained high or low glucose levels, go into troubleshooting mode. Check infusion sites, the tubing, the reservoir, the insulin (it may have expired or been exposed to excessive heat or cold), your pump settings, your recent insulin delivery history, and whether the pump is properly functioning.

➡ It is important for someone using insulin pump therapy to understand that he or she can develop ketones if the pump stops delivering insulin. Because you no longer have long-acting or basal insulin in your body, ketones may form as soon as 3 hours after the insulin infusion is interrupted. You develop ketones when you do not have enough insulin in the bloodstream—even if you have been taking your usual doses but it doesn't meet your metabolic needs. Ketones develop with infection, stress, or illness. Most frequently, hyperglycemia and ketones go hand in hand, but you may have only mild hyperglycemia, a normal glucose level, or even a low glucose level and still have ketones.

➡ You need to work with your diabetes team and other health care providers to know what to do with your insulin pump if you are hospitalized.

➡ If your pump stops working, it might take a day or two to get a replacement pump. You can manage your diabetes with rapid-acting insulin only. Calculate your meal and correction boluses the same way you would if you were still on your pump. For your basal rate, you will need to calculate how much insulin you need to take every 2 or 3 hours to replace your basal rate and then determine how much to give as injections. You might want to replace your basal insulin with a shot of long-acting insulin every 12 or 24 hours.

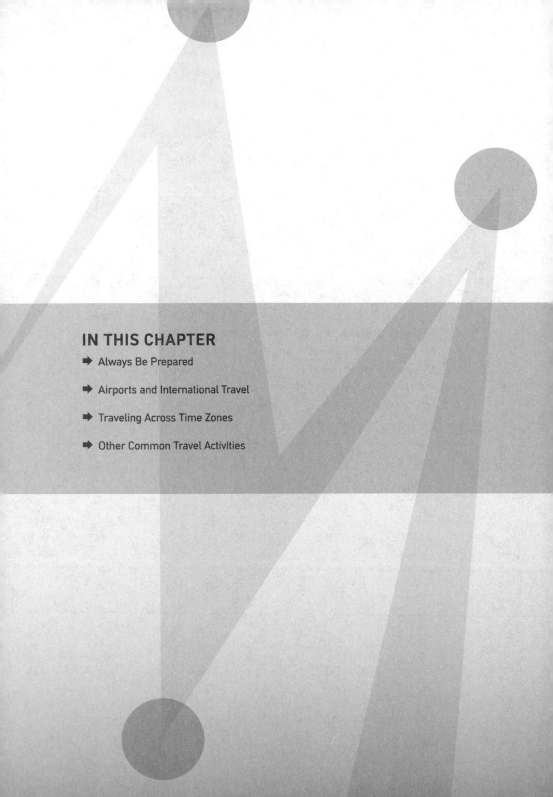

IN THIS CHAPTER

CHAPTER 14

TRAVEL WITH THE PUMP AND A CGM

Traveling with diabetes requires planning, and traveling with the pump and a continuous glucose monitor (CGM) requires even a bit more planning. The good news is that the pump and CGM allow for easy adjustments and will likely give you better diabetes control while you travel. You can adjust your basal rates, alter your boluses, and adjust the clock on the pump. You can adjust your insulin administration if you are increasing or decreasing your activity levels during specific parts of the day (e.g., walking around a big city, hiking or backpacking, or being sedentary on road trips). You can easily give yourself correction boluses for foreign foods or if you're treating yourself to local snacks and desserts (like crepes in France or gelato in Italy). While wearing the CGM, you can be alerted to rapid and potentially dangerous fluctuations in your glucose levels as the result of the change in your routine and your sleeping patterns. You can alter your alerts (raise the low alert and lower the high alert) to be notified of glucose changes earlier so that you can be proactive and take action.

There are a few key things that you must always remember when traveling while on the pump and CGM. By arming yourself with knowledge and by being prepared, worldwide travel will be what you always dreamed it would be.

ALWAYS BE PREPARED

Travel requires extra vigilance with diabetes management, no matter which therapy you are using. Crossing time zones, sampling new foods, frequent changes in activity level, and the everyday stress of travel (airport security, rushing to catch a train, or waiting in endless lines) can all affect your glucose levels. The number one rule for safe travel is to check your glucose levels frequently. This step is best accomplished with a CGM. And always be prepared to treat a low or high glucose level by having extra glucose tablets, food, or juice with you at all times, along with your insulin and diabetes supplies.

When you are on MDI, you must always have adequate amounts of extra insulin and syringes with you when you travel. This is a good idea if you're leaving town even for the day. With the pump and CGM, it is a good idea to bring a few more things with you, including syringes and extra insulin in case there is an issue with your pump. Below is a list of the items that you should always have in a backpack or travel kit for any kind of travel.

- **Pump emergency card.** This is a card given to you by most pump companies. It has your name, your device name and details, and treatment recommendations should something happen to you. This information can also come from your health care team.

- **Extra infusion sets and extra sensors.** Pack two or more, depending on how long you'll be gone. If the infusion set you're using when you leave fails and then for some reason your backup fails too, then you will still have a backup. When you travel for more than a few nights, you might want to think of bringing two sets for every 3 days of travel. The same goes for sensors. Pack extras in case you need to remove a sensor earlier than expected. Depending on the length of time you are gone (a couple weeks to months, for example), you might want to think of bringing an extra transmitter as well. It may seem like a lot, but it's better to be prepared than to be without a set or a sensor.

  —For every infusion set you bring, you'll also want to bring a reservoir. You might not need quite as many reservoirs because they usually aren't the parts that malfunction.

- **Syringes or insulin pens.** A couple of syringes will be necessary if you are in a situation where you are unable to change a set and your glucose levels are inexplicably high. Syringes are also necessary if you develop ketones. You could opt to carry insulin pens (and pen needles) with rapid-acting insulin if you'd rather pack those than syringes and vials.

- **Extra vial(s) of rapid-acting insulin.** If you are gone for longer than 1–2 weeks, you might want to think about taking two vials. This is especially important if you are traveling somewhere abroad and are unable to get your prescriptions filled easily if something goes wrong.

- **A vial or pen of basal insulin.** If you are comfortable using long-acting insulins or happen to have some on hand, bring them with you while traveling in case you need to return to MDI therapy.

- **Extra strips.** You will always need extra test strips when traveling. Even if you use a CGM, you want to be sure you have enough strips in case your sensor falls off early, for while you are on the plane, and because you will likely need to correct and adjust your insulin more often.

  — If you're going abroad, it's wise to bring another blood glucose meter, lancing device with lancets, and batteries. These will be needed if any part of your current kit fails or if you want to leave a kit in your room and have one to take on outings.

- **Extra tape for infusion sets and sensors, appropriate fluids or wipes, and other application or removal aids.** Basically, the rule

TRAVELING WITH INSULIN

- Insulin must have a current prescription label on the box. This will prove that you have a justifiable reason for carrying all your other medical equipment and syringes.
- Be sure that the insulin has not expired.
- If you are traveling for an extended period of time, think about bringing a cooler and cooling pack.

is "If you use it at home, bring it along." If you use a preparation to remove tape adhesive or to protect your sites at home, then you're going to want it when you're traveling. Also, bringing extra tape is a good idea even if you don't normally use it. Vacationing and traveling often throw you into situations where your tubing could get pulled out, your sets could be damaged, or your sensors fall off—particularly if you are in water all day. That little bit of extra security tape might just save you from having a pulled-off sensor, with loss of your glucose tracing, or a dislodged catheter, causing a high glucose level.

- **Extra batteries.** Make sure you have extra batteries for your pump as well as for your test kit (and your CGM, if you have one). You don't want to go searching for batteries on your vacation. Keeping a few handy will guarantee that you won't be stuck with a pump and no means to power it.

- **A way to safely dispose of sharps.** It might be inconvenient to bring your small sharps container or some other container to safely dispose of your used needles, but it is important. Don't forget—safety precautions should be followed everywhere. There are small needle clippers that you can buy at local pharmacies. These are compact and remove needles to the base of the syringe or pen needle. This device is tamper-proof and allows you to throw away the syringe once the needle is fully removed. Once full, dispose of it as you would with other biohazards and sharps.

- **Ketone testing equipment.** Whether it is foil-wrapped strips, a vial, or a blood ketone monitor, you must have a way to check for ketones when traveling.

- **Glucagon.** Transportation Security Administration (TSA) officials may check your bag of supplies. It is easiest to explain if there is a prescription label on the glucagon kit. Be sure it has not expired.

- **Food, glucose tabs, etc.** Be sure to have food, glucose tabs, glucose gel, or whatever you need to treat low glucose levels.

- **Loaner or travel pump.** Some companies will send you an extra insulin pump as a "travel pump" in case something happens to yours while you are away. It can cost around $50 and, for some companies, must be insured. But this extra pump can be a lifesaver if yours breaks, is misplaced, or is stolen. These pumps are usually only available for international travel because you can get a pump within 24 hours if you are still in the U.S.

AIRPORTS AND INTERNATIONAL TRAVEL

International air travel with medical devices can be difficult if security personnel are not familiar with insulin pumps and CGMs. Give yourself plenty of time before your flight leaves so you don't miss it if you are delayed for security reasons. It is important to have the printed prescription labels for all of your diabetes supplies with you when you travel. The prescription labels can be taken off insulin boxes, the box for your insulin syringes, and the box for your pump supplies and placed in a bag or other container. The prescription labels must match your name on your identification, such as your driver's license or passport. A note from the doctor on official stationery might also be helpful. However, because these are so easily forged, it is more important to show that you have prescriptions for all of your medications.

Other countries have different electric plug outlets and electrical current capacities. If your diabetes devices have batteries that are charged every few days, make sure to bring the appropriate converter. Also, consider whether your CGM transmits to your phone. You should be able to use your phone on Bluetooth-only mode or turn off roaming to not use data in other countries. Transmission to a cloud or sharing system may require Wi-Fi or a data plan.

SEPARATE YOUR INSULIN VIALS

Sometimes it is smart to put a vial of insulin in a different location, so if one of them gets lost or is ruined by heat or cold, you still have another good one.

NO X-RAYS FOR YOUR DEVICES

Your pump and CGM should NOT go through the X-ray machine. However, they can pass through the metal detector.

You might be stopped if you have a CGM and it has a separate receiver. Neither the pump nor the receiver should go through the X-ray machine. This usually means that security staff will need to inspect you by hand. Often, they will do a search or swab all of your carry-ons and do a pat-down. If you choose to go the route of pat-down and hand inspection, plan for this to take around 30 extra minutes. Sometimes, TSA will only do a hand-swab of you and your devices.

Talk to your health care team before you plan on leaving the country, because they may be able to tell you how to manage prescriptions or emergencies in other countries. Another helpful contact is your health insurance company. Health insurance representatives may be able to assist you in finding places where you can buy supplies or insulin. Some companies make pumps, sensors, and supplies that have similar names in other countries, but they may not work with U.S. pumps and CGM systems. Before you leave home, it may be helpful to know whether your supplies are compatible with the other country's supplies in case of an emergency.

If you are worried about communication problems with security personnel abroad, you might want to translate your doctor's note or other important information into that country's language before you leave.

TRAVELING ACROSS TIME ZONES

If you're traveling across time zones, you will likely experience jet lag. Jet lag not only means difficulty adjusting to a new sleeping pattern; it also means your body has to change its metabolic and hormone secretion patterns that are associated with your sleep/wake cycles. Your liver releases stored glucose at different rates depending on whether you are awake or asleep. Adjusting your basal rates can really help with glucose control when you are jet lagged.

If you're taking a short or long trip or anything in between, then you can probably just change your pump and CGM time during travel to the time at your destination (for example, if you're going from Los Angeles to New York, a 3-hour time change, then you can just change the time on your pump and CGM during your flight or once you land). If you are crossing multiple time zones (from New York to Australia), you may need a day or two before your sleep-wake cycles regulate. Also, your basal rates may not easily translate from one time zone to the next. Think about when your basal rates are the highest at home (normally in the daytime) and when that higher basal rate will fall when you land and reset the time on your pump. If you travel around the world, this may swap your highest and lowest basal rates, causing highs and lows in your glucose levels until you acclimate to the new time zone. Be sure to watch your CGM or test frequently to avoid these issues.

Your goal should be to establish your sleep/wake cycle to match where you are, and this is the same goal for your basal rate timing as well. Check more often to be sure.

Long-Term Travel (Study Abroad or Volunteer Activities)

At some point in your life, you may decide to travel for longer than a week or two. This may be for a school opportunity (study abroad or a school tour) or for an elongated trip abroad (a vacation or a volunteer opportunity). In these events, you must plan ahead and potentially stock up on your supplies so that you don't run out while away. If you will be gone longer than 1 month and your prescriptions normally come in a single-month supply, you may need to have your health care team write a prescription for 3 months or call your insurance company and discuss your options. Consider how much room your supplies will take up. They may require an entire suitcase if you are gone for several months. You will need to think about everything that you may need at some point and pack extras on top of that. You can buy AA and AAA batteries in most countries, but it is a good idea to bring some along in case you can't find any.

OTHER COMMON TRAVEL ACTIVITIES

It's common to exercise more when you travel. Watch your basal rates and glucose levels closely and always bring extra food in case you go low. Glucose tabs are surprisingly difficult to find abroad or even in some places in the U.S., so bringing a good supply with you is a smart idea. Bring enough treatments for hypoglycemia so you can treat yourself until you find something to buy locally (candy like Skittles™ works in a pinch). Another good idea is to bring snack bars or some kind of snack that has starch and protein so you always have enough glucose in your blood. These are nice also for "meals" in airports or for times when you're unable to find food and you need to eat.

Camping and Skiing

When camping, you need to consider altitude, temperature, physical activity, and food supply. Be sure you can control the temperatures to which the insulin in your pump, your extra insulin vials, and other critical supplies are exposed. If you are carrying these supplies with you at all times, you might want to think about getting temperature-controlled packs for cooling and protective covering to avoid freezing. A small lunchbox with an ice pack can keep your insulin and supplies at acceptable temperatures for a few days, as long as it is not placed in direct sunlight (this might turn it into a small oven!). In freezing weather, keep your pump, tubing, CGM receiver, and supplies inside your coat and next to your body, where they will be kept warm. (This also applies if you live somewhere with harsh winters.)

Altitude changes can create air bubbles or increase their frequency, so check your tubing often. Altitude, exercise, and camping food can also affect the amount of insulin you need. Altitude can also affect sleeping patterns, which in turn can affect the amount of insulin you need. When you go up in elevation, there is less oxygen in the air you are breathing. Your breathing will increase as your body works harder to produce the same amount of energy with less oxygen. Things that aren't difficult at your normal elevation will be much harder (such as climbing stairs and brisk walking). As your body works harder, it may require more glucose and can cause low glucose levels. On the other hand, for some people, high altitude acts more like a stress and produces stress hormones that cause high glucose levels.

Altitude sickness is also very hard on the body. When you get altitude sickness, you may get a headache, lose your appetite, or vomit. These are all side effects of not getting enough oxygen. If you begin to vomit or feel nauseated, test ketones and treat this like a sick day. Come down in elevation if you can. Because of your increased breathing rate, you will exhale more water and the climate will likely be dry. Therefore, it is important to stay hydrated. Drink more!

Talk to your diabetes team about reducing your basal rates and boluses, when to suspend, and how to adjust your doses as your trip progresses. Don't forget to check your glucose often and in the middle of the night to reduce your risk of severe hypoglycemia. If you have a CGM, make sure it is calibrated and reading accurately so that you can determine if your insulin requirements are changing.

Beach Days

When you go to the beach, you will need to plan on disconnecting from your pump and consider your activity level and how you will protect your pump, CGM controller, and infusion set from heat, sand, and water. Everyone knows that sand gets everywhere and can disrupt your insulin pump and insertion sites. If you remove your pump, think about placing it in a plastic bag in a cooler. This protects it from sand and keeps your insulin from overheating in the sun. Remember, ice packs can freeze insulin if they are in direct contact—this should be avoided. Also be careful not to submerge your pump in water unless you are sure it is waterproof and free of cracks and scratches.

Most infusion sets come with clip-on safety covers for the insertion site. These are handy because sand will creep into the attachment's crevices and prevent a complete connection when you decide to put your pump back on or when you take a correction bolus. Although, you don't have to worry about sand or seawater getting into your body when you're swimming, even if you don't have the safety cover. These sets are designed to let in only insulin via the tubing, and the catheter will not let in water, other liquids, or sand. It should also be noted that the safety cover will not prevent a set from being pulled out, so bring an extra couple of sets. As always, check your blood glucose often to be sure you won't spoil a great beach day with fluctuating glucose levels.

Amusement Parks

A day at the amusement park can be harder to manage than you might think. You need to consider the temperature, your activity level, hydration, food choices, and a whole lot of adrenaline. Waiting in long lines in the sun can lead to overheating—of you, your pump, and your insulin. Standing in long lines in the sun can cause hypoglycemia, but if your insulin overheats you may become hyperglycemic. See if the park has a program for people with special needs; this might help reduce the time you spend waiting in lines. Watch your food choices, as these foods often contain more carbohydrates, more fat, and have larger portion sizes than you might normally eat. Drink plenty of water, check your glucose levels often (particularly after you have been screaming on rides that turn you upside down and have you going at extraordinary speeds). Under these conditions, anything can happen to your glucose levels, so be cautious. Don't overcorrect those highs from an adrenaline rush. They usually don't last very long. Consider a way to secure your meter, pump, CGM receiver, and other supplies for these rides (such as a fanny pack). You don't want your supplies to fly out of your pockets on rides with high speeds and loops.

Are We There Yet? Long Trips by Car, Plane, Boat, or Train

When you are traveling a long distance over a long time period, consider what happens when you get almost no exercise. During long trips, you get less exercise than usual, even if you have a desk job. You hardly move your muscles. In turn, your muscles don't use much glucose, possibly causing your insulin requirements to increase. For long road trips, you might need to increase your basal rates or take more insulin for your correction and food boluses. This is a good time to consider a temporary increase in basal rates, by 10–20% initially (110–120% basal rate), and then increase as needed depending on your glucose levels.

Watch your food choices for your snacks and meals. We all know that road trips, train stations, and airports are filled with less-than-healthy food choices. Combined with lack of activity, these foods might increase your glucose to a higher number faster than usual. Look at your CGM tracing, or test your blood glucose often, bolus before you eat, and drink plenty of fluids to help manage your glucose levels during your travels.

CHAPTER REVIEW

➡ Travel requires extra vigilance. Crossing time zones, eating new foods, changing activity levels, and the everyday stresses of travel can all affect your glucose levels. The first rule for safe travel is to check your glucose levels frequently and to be prepared at all times to treat with extra food or insulin.

➡ Getting through the airport can be difficult. Be prepared for delays at security and know that your pump and CGM should not go through the X-ray machine. But these devices can pass through the metal detector.

➡ Crossing time zones can be difficult for anyone. Your goal should be to establish your sleep/wake pattern to match where you are, and this is the same goal for your basal rate timing as well.

➡ Doing everything everyone else does should be your goal. Being prepared—having sufficient supplies, checking glucose levels often, and factoring in your activity level—will help you have safe diabetes management wherever you go.

IN THIS CHAPTER

- Your Personal Diabetes Medical Management Plan
- The Pump or CGM in the Classroom
- College with an Insulin Pump

CHAPTER 15

THE PUMP AT SCHOOL: FROM THE BEGINNING THROUGH COLLEGE

Diabetes must be managed 24 hours a day, 7 days a week. This means that diabetes must be effectively managed at school, too. Because careful monitoring of glucose levels must occur throughout the school day and insulin must be administered, it is important to have coordination and collaboration between the students, parents, school nurses, teachers, school administrators, and diabetes health care team. This process is best accomplished through meetings, familiarity with regulations, and a written diabetes management plan, regardless of whether the student uses an insulin pump or injection therapy. By following these steps, the student with diabetes can be safe, have optimal diabetes management, and be able to have a positive and rewarding school experience.

School personnel—most importantly the school nurse and teachers—must understand the basics of diabetes as well as of insulin pump therapy. You need to understand your rights under the Americans with Disabilities Act. Together, you must devise the plan that allows for you or your child to be effectively and safely managed in school.

There are valuable resources available. Visit the Safe at School page on the American Diabetes Association's website (www.diabetes.org/safeatschool). Be sure to also read *Helping the Student with Diabetes Succeed: A Guide for School Personnel*, which is available on the National Diabetes Education Program website (https://www.niddk.nih.gov/health-information/health-communication-programs/ndep/health-care-professionals/school-guide/section3/Documents/NDEP-School-Guide-Full.pdf).

YOUR PERSONAL DIABETES MEDICAL MANAGEMENT PLAN

There are three management plans that you must devise for the school. They outline exactly what is required for success with diabetes and insulin pump therapy.

1. **Diabetes Medical Management Plan (DMMP).** The DMMP is completed by the student's diabetes health care team and contains the medical orders that are the basis for the student's health care and education plans.

2. **Individualized Health Plan (IHP).** This plan is developed by the school nurse in collaboration with the student's diabetes health care team and family to put the medical recommendations in the student's DMMP into practice in the school.

3. **Emergency care plans for hypoglycemia and hyperglycemia.** These emergency care plans are based on the medical orders, summarize how to recognize and treat hypoglycemia and hyperglycemia, and describe whom to contact for help. These plans, developed by the school nurse, should be distributed to all school personnel who are responsible for the student with diabetes during the school day and during school-sponsored activities.

The DMMP is set up between your diabetes care team, the school nurse, and you (and your child). The school will require a written assessment of the child's diabetes health. It will cover all of the actions required for blood glucose testing, continuous glucose monitor (CGM) calibrations and alerts, treating hypoglycemia and hyperglycemia, eating, exercising, ketone testing, field trips, delivery of boluses, pump disconnections, who is to treat the student in emergencies, and any other necessary medical information about managing glucose levels (this includes the child's ability to treat himself or herself independently, other medications, mental conditions, and hypoglycemia unawareness). The DMMP must be absolutely accurate, updated often, and always available, since the nurse will use this to determine the IHP's strategies for

Members of the School Health Team	Members of the Student's Diabetes Health Care Team
Student with diabetes	Student with diabetes
Parent(s)/guardian	Parent(s)/guardian
School nurse	Doctor
Other school health care personnel	Nurse
Trained diabetes personnel	Registered dietitian
Administrators	Diabetes educator
Principal	Other health care providers involved with
504 Plan/Individualized Education Plan (IEP) coordinator	the student's diabetes care
Office staff	
Student's teacher(s)	
Guidance counselor	
Coach, lunchroom and other school staff	

diabetes care at school and a 504 Plan or Individualized Education Plan (IEP), if used (covered under Federal Laws, later in this chapter).

A DMMP should include details about the child's overall diabetes care and CGM and pump use. It is a guideline and is meant to provide instructions for common concerns or issues that are related to diabetes. There is no way to predict everything that might happen, and the DMMP should not be viewed as a complete, inflexible instruction manual. Parents or guardians can override the DMMP if they need to, and they should always be contacted if there are any questions or concerns about a child's treatment.

Here is a list of information that should always be included in the DMMP. Sample forms for a DMMP are available on the websites noted in this section.

- **Child's information.** Include child's name, date of birth, classroom/grade, address, home phone, and parent/guardian's cell or work phone.

- **Current diabetes information.** Include date of diagnosis, current A1C, level of diabetes awareness (a younger child's ability to recognize high or low glucose levels, an older child's independent abilities, knowledge of the pump's capabilities, how to use and calibrate a CGM, and any automated insulin delivery features, etc.), overall diabetes health, types of insulins used, and the brand, serial number, and model names for the blood glucose meter, insulin pump, and CGM. The phone number for the help line for the pump and CGM device should also be included.

- **Diabetes doctor's contact information.** Include doctor's name, phone number, and location of practice. Include this information for other health care providers, such as nurses, physician assistants, and nurse practitioners.

- **Emergency contact information.** The emergency contact might include another guardian, a separate family member, or a friend who can also assist in case of an emergency if you cannot be reached.

- **Specific instructions.** These instructions will change depending on the child's age and capabilities with his or her own diabetes care. This section should be updated often and will include:

  —*Assistance with glucose monitoring, CGM calibration and alerts, any automated insulin delivery features, and logging.* Who can assist with glucose monitoring, where that assistance will be done, how the child/assistant will respond to alarms and perform calibrations, and what information gets recorded needs to be defined. Have your diabetes care team discuss the ability to use CGM for dosing at school if that is indicated with your CGM.

  —*Instructions for hypoglycemia.* Definition of and treatment for mild, moderate, and severe lows. When and how to disconnect the pump.

  —*Instructions for hyperglycemia.* List the child's insulin sensitivity factor, describe whether insulin is to be given by pump or syringe, detail ketone testing, and indicate when infusion sets should be changed.

— *How and when to administer glucagon.*

— *How and when to check for ketones.*

— *Instructions for meal and snack boluses.* List the child's carbohydrate ratios. Define who counts the carbs, who enters them into the pump, and who approves giving insulin. Also note whether a dual-wave or square-wave bolus should be used for specific foods and how that is done.

— *Pump storage.*

— *Temporary basal rates for physical activity (if needed).*

— *CGM care and usage.* Describe when a calibration is needed and how to do it.

— *How to change an infusion set.* Describe how to fill the reservoir, prime the tubing, and connect and fill the cannula.

- **All medications kept and administered at school.** These include insulin and any other medications, for diabetes or other conditions.

- **Typical symptoms.** Symptoms for both hypoglycemia and hyperglycemia should be covered, and it should be indicated whether the child is able to recognize the symptoms.

- **List of supplies and equipment worn and used daily.** This list might also include what the child should keep at school as well as which supplies are kept in each room/area (e.g., supplies for changing sets, sensors, and insulin in the nurse's office; ketone testing equipment; blood glucose test kit and treatment for hypoglycemia in the classroom and treatment for hypoglycemia in a gym locker or with the gym teacher).

- **Special field trips and excursion instructions.**

- **Sharps and sharps disposal.**

- **Other medical information.** Include allergies, other conditions (such as celiac disease), mental diagnosis, and psychological diagnosis.

MANAGING YOUR DMMP

An updated copy of the DMMP should be kept with the school nurse, homeroom teacher, and parents at all times. In the beginning of every year or when something changes in your child's plan, the DMMP should be revised, reviewed, and signed by all necessary individuals (this might include a diabetes educator, a school administrator, the guardians, a school nurse, and the homeroom teacher).

Federal Laws

You should familiarize yourself with the three federal laws that address the school's responsibilities to help students with diabetes: Section 504 of the Rehabilitation Act of 1973 (Section 504), the Americans with Disabilities Act of 1990 (ADA), and the Individuals with Disabilities Education Act (IDEA). These federal laws provide a framework for planning and implementing effective diabetes management in the school setting, for preparing the student's education plan, and for protecting the student's privacy. The requirements of federal laws must always be met. School administrators and nursing personnel should determine whether applicable state and local laws need to be factored into helping students with diabetes.

The school will work with you to meet the federal regulations. Your child should develop a 504 Plan or an IEP to ensure that his or her medical and academic needs will be met. The 504 Plan sets out an agreement to make sure the student with diabetes has the same access to education as other children. Students who qualify for services under IDEA will have an IEP instead of a 504 Plan. Typically, an IEP is more specific and focused than a 504 Plan, detailing the student's academic needs, current level of functioning, supports, and goals.

THE PUMP OR CGM IN THE CLASSROOM

You must determine where you or your child will do glucose monitoring. It is best—if you and your child agree—to check blood and sensor glucose levels and treat them within the classroom, anytime and anywhere. Leaving the classroom to go to the nurse's office or elsewhere means that the child may be without supervision while going to check, that there could be a delay in finding and treating high and low glucose levels, and that classroom time and instruction will be missed. You also need to consider where you want bolus insulin administration to occur: in the classroom, the lunchroom, or someplace else, such as the nurse's office. Finally, you need to consider where you want infusion set and sensor changes to occur and other medications given, likely not in the classroom. Allowing diabetes tasks (particularly with the pump and the sensor) to occur anytime and anyplace helps normalize these procedures as well as improve the skills of the child.

Teachers, substitutes, and other school personnel (principals, counselors, etc.) should be aware that the pump or CGM receiver is not a game. They also need to know that your child may also need to carry a cell phone if it serves as a receiver, a way to transmit data, or if it is used to discuss management issues with a parent.

It may be helpful for you to set up time with teachers and administrators to let them hear the alarms and to understand what your child may need to do to respond to them. It will reduce the knee-jerk reaction teachers may have to reprimand an audible alarm. If a teacher knows the sound of a low glucose alarm, a low reservoir, or a predicted high glucose alarm, it will help them address it appropriately and make sure that the alarm is not disruptive to the class. It may also be helpful to have a discussion between the child/family and teacher concerning where the child will keep the pump/CGM so the devices can be checked during class.

INDEPENDENCE AND CONFIDENCE

The ability to test and treat in the classroom, lunchroom, gymnasium, and elsewhere makes checking glucose (either by blood or sensor) a normal part of the school day. When a child is allowed to test and treat in the classroom, the child with diabetes as well as his or her peers will view these as regular activities.

It is likely even more important to meet with school personnel about cell phones. Because more and more diabetes devices are being transmitted to cell phones, it is important to inform the school that these phones must be allowed. All school personnel need to know they cannot confiscate them. And you need to have a discussion with your child to be sure they don't abuse the privilege or use it for anything other than diabetes.

Security When Disconnecting

During class, if the student needs to disconnect the pump for a time, there needs to be a designated area to safely store the pump that is in a cool, dry place and that can be secured so that the pump cannot be taken or tampered with. There also needs to be a place for the receiver of the CGM, if there is one. For gym class, if the DMMP designates disconnecting the pump, a locker that can be secured, the gym teacher's office, or the nurse's office are good choices for safe storage. Unfortunately, pumps, glucose meters, and other diabetes equipment can be stolen.

Field Trips

No child should be prohibited from a school activity because of diabetes. However, special considerations need to be in place to ensure that there is adequate supervision for diabetes management and the pump. This supervision may include having the responsible adult agree to respond to parents who are viewing their child's CGM remotely.

Meal and Snack Time

It is the obligation of the school to provide nutrition information for the foods offered. With appropriate nutrition information, the child (if he or she is capable) or the responsible adult in the school can ensure that the correct amount of insulin is taken. Other foods such as snacks and treats that are not part of the school's official meal policies should have nutrition information made available if possible. It is a common requirement that any treats brought in from

Teaching your child how to read a nutrition label early will help them become independent and feel good about taking control of their diabetes.

outside are prepackaged and not made at home. These foods should have a nutrition label.

School Schedule

The school schedule, with regard to meals, snacks, gym class, and recess, should be discussed by the parents and school personnel. Adjustments in the diabetes regimen—and the school schedule, if needed—should be made to help the child successfully manage blood glucose levels. If each semester has a different daily schedule, the DMMP may need to be altered to accommodate the activity changes.

Extra Supplies

Extra supplies should always be kept at school. There should be enough to last 72 hours, in case there is a natural disaster or an emergency that lasts a few days. Supplies should be stored in a secure area but should also be easily accessible. Most often, they are kept in the nurse's office. If a child needs to use an infusion set or other supplies from the supply cache, be aware that these supplies need to be replenished to remain properly stocked. Check in with the nurse every few weeks to make sure that there is always the proper amount of supplies. Supplies should include the following:

- Insulin (rapid- and perhaps long-acting)
- Syringes and/or pen needles
- Infusion sets
- Reservoirs
- Tape

- Adhesive aids and/or removing agents

- Numbing agents that the child uses for a new sensor or infusion set insertion

- Extra blood glucose monitor and lancet

- Extra test strips

- Extra lancets

- Batteries or charging cables for the pump, blood glucose meter, and CGM

- Any insertion device needed for infusion sets or syringes

- Urine ketone strips or blood ketone monitor

- Fast-acting carbohydrates (such as juice, glucose tabs, or glucose gel) and snacks with protein (such as peanut butter or cheese crackers or granola bars) for treating low glucose levels

- Glucagon

- Emergency contact information and doctor's information

- Extra sensors if you are comfortable with your child inserting sensors without supervision

Discussing the Pump at School

For elementary school children, diabetes and the insulin pump and CGM can awaken curiosity. Friends and classmates often want to ask many questions, touch the pump or sensor, and figure out what it does. As long as it is okay with the child, arrange a "show-and-tell" about diabetes, the pump, and the sensor. It is important, however, to make sure that your child feels safe and comfortable with the idea of a presentation because many children are shy about their diabetes. If a show-and-tell introduction to the class is embarrassing for your child, discuss how he or she would like to deal with curious classmates. One option is to write a letter that goes home with classmates. By preparing children for these types of scenarios, you may be able to teach them more about diabetes, and they might acquire a sense of pride when they can explain what diabetes is and how the pump and sensor helps them live a normal life.

Special Accommodations

During school examinations, your child will still need access to testing equipment, a source of glucose, and insulin via the pump. Accommodations for this step should be discussed before exams begin. The student might be placed in a separate room and should be allowed to manage his or her diabetes without that influencing the exam results. For timed examinations, the time needed to check glucose levels and possibly correct them should not be counted.

These considerations can be incorporated into the 504 Plan but must be decided and arranged before the testing. By arranging any specific testing accommodations (e.g., necessary supplies or changing testing times based on glucose levels being out of range) at the beginning of the year, the teachers and child know what actions are to be made regarding testing. Administration won't take kindly to a child needing a different testing schedule because of glucose levels or children who need their diabetes technology with them in a test (such as the SAT or ACT) when there were no prior discussions. Standardized testing policies are very strict about devices being allowed during test taking. A 504 Plan will ensure your child can bring in their supplies/devices (glucose, glucose meter, pump, and CGM receiver), but they may not be allowed to use a phone for a CGM receiver. If your child is taking standardized tests, be sure to research policies and start any special requests or accommodations early to ensure they are allowed.

Further Resources

- The American Diabetes Association's website covering discrimination at school and work has several helpful articles on the topic (http://www.diabetes.org/living-with-diabetes/parents-and-kids/diabetes-care-at-school/medical-scientific-sources-authority.html).

- The National Diabetes Education Program has a book that provides sample DMMPs and other forms for schools, parents, and students. It is called *Helping the Student with Diabetes Succeed: A Guide for School Personnel* and is available at https://www.niddk.nih.gov/health-information/health-communication-programs/ndep/health-care-professionals/school-guide/section3/Documents/NDEP-School-Guide-Full.pdf.

- Contact the pump company if you have questions about integrating the pump into the school environment. These companies have a 24-hour helpline that may be a good resource when putting together presentations for classmates, school personnel, or teachers. Pump manufacturers can also provide specific pump information for the DMMP.

COLLEGE WITH AN INSULIN PUMP

Having an insulin pump and CGM during college can help manage the ups and downs, crazy schedules, fast food, stress, and all the other things that college life involves. CGM alerts can be used to alert you about all those glucose ups and downs. If you know how to use your pump's key features and have good knowledge of how your body reacts to different treatments, then you have the resources to succeed with the pump and CGM during school.

Even without diabetes, college is a turbulent time that will force you to adapt and roll with the punches. Sports, classes, tests, homework, on-campus dining (and off-campus dining, for that matter), dorm life, new places, and new people will all affect glucose and diabetes care. It can be tricky, but, when used properly, the pump and CGM can be useful tools to get you through college with good glucose levels. The grades are up to you.

The Schedule That Isn't One

For many students in college, their schedule varies from day to day. Some days require getting up much earlier than others, and some days require sitting in several classes back-to-back with no breaks for meals. It is a good idea to check basal rates before attending college to determine if they are appropriate. After getting your class schedule, think about how to prepare for different days. Maybe 3 of the 5 days include a sport; you might want to make a new basal pattern for those days. Do you have four back-to-back classes that prohibit lunch? For those days, making sure you have adequate snacks is important, or you should pack a lunch to eat on the go. Unexpected schedule disruptions like long study sessions often include lots of snacking, which can increase your blood glucose. Make sure you administer sufficient insulin to cover these snacks. Stress may also play a role in your diabetes management.

Alcohol

Alcohol can be found on almost any college campus—despite the fact that underage drinking is illegal. Alcohol affects glucose levels and can lead to severe hypoglycemia.

When alcohol is ingested, it decreases the ability of the liver to release stored glucose. If a large amount of alcohol is ingested without food, particularly before bedtime, there is the risk of severe hypoglycemia during sleep and even the next day. Therefore, if you decide to drink, plan on reducing insulin doses, checking glucose often if you self-monitor blood glucose, wearing your CGM with the low alert set higher (or using the automated insulin suspension set higher), eating, and being sure someone around you knows that you have diabetes.

The best plan, however, is never to drink if you are not an adult and never to drink in excess if you are an adult. For adults, drinking in excess is defined as more than 1 drink a day for women and as more than 2 drinks a day for men.

Your Dorm, Your Resident Assistant, and Your Roommate

Having a roommate or roommates is part of college life. When you're getting to know each other, you should tell your roommate about your diabetes. At a minimum, he or she needs to know about hypoglycemia, what you will look and act like, what he or she can do to help (if you want help), and when to call 911 if you are unresponsive or confused.

In addition, tell your roommates about the pump. Explain what it does and that you will almost always be wearing it. Show them your CGM and how it sends glucose information to the pump screen or receiver. Answer any questions they might have. If you share a refrigerator, let them know that your insulin is what keeps you alive and that it is not to be tampered with; the same goes for your supplies for glucose monitoring and for the pump. Also assure them that you will follow the universal safety precautions for your sharps from the infusion set, lancets, and syringes. The more you can tell them, the safer your living situation will be. You must also tell the resident assistant in your dorm that you have diabetes and inform him or her of what should be done in an emergency. Of course, you should consider sharing the fact that you have diabetes with new friends as well. Sometimes a written document that describes where supplies are located and how to treat diabetes emergencies (such as how to administer glucagon) is helpful for roommates and hall directors.

Health Services
You should go to health services when you arrive on campus. Let them know that you have diabetes and that you use an insulin pump and a CGM. Give them information about your diabetes history, your present insulin doses, and your overall management plan. Give them the names and numbers of your diabetes team and make them a part of the network of your diabetes care providers.

Running Out of Supplies
For some, going to college means that they will be in charge of their supplies for the first time. Parents can't always check in to remind you about reordering your supplies. Discussing how to refill prescriptions for pump supplies, insulin, sensors and other CGM supplies, and test strips is vital. Sit down and brainstorm ways to remember to reorder your supplies. If you are left with only one or two infusion sets or sensors, you will not have enough time to refill your order by mail. Try imposing the "last box" rule. Whenever you

notice you are about to open your last box of supplies, you order more—right away. If you are a procrastinator, use the "second-to-last-box" rule. Do a test run of ordering supplies before leaving for college so you are comfortable with this routine.

CHAPTER REVIEW

➡ A DMMP should include details about the child's overall diabetes care, CGM, and pump use. It is a guideline and is meant to serve as instructions for common concerns or issues related to diabetes at school.

➡ The ability to test and treat in the classroom, lunchroom, gymnasium, and other places makes checking glucose (either by blood or sensor) and diabetes management a normal part of the school day. The child with diabetes as well as his or her peers will view managing diabetes as a regular activity.

➡ Having an insulin pump and CGM during college can help manage the ups and downs, crazy schedules, fast food, stress, and all the other things that college life involves.

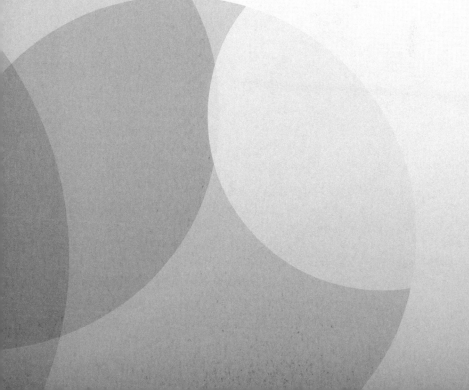

SECTION 5:
ADJUSTING TO INSULIN PUMP AND CGM THERAPIES

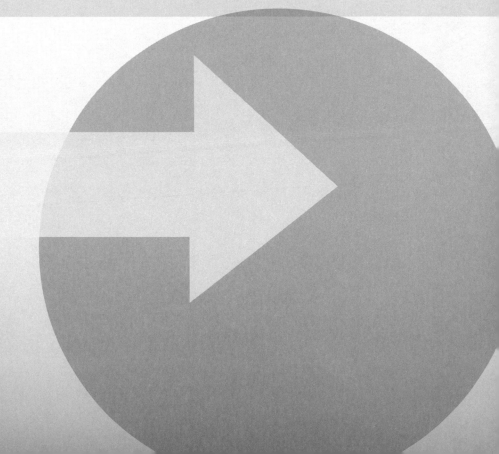

CHAPTER 16

CAPABILITIES BY AGE

Depending on your age (or your child's age), some tasks for diabetes management and pump therapy will require assistance. The assistance can be in the form of either technical or cognitive assistance. But remember, it is always important that someone stays involved, is aware of how diabetes control is progressing, and is there to offer help (e.g., to ask about glucose control and overall psychological adjustment). Diabetes is just too big—even for the most capable adult—to deal with alone.

DEVELOPMENT AND COGNITIVE SKILLS BY AGE RANGE

Helping your child develop the skills and confidence necessary to assume age-appropriate responsibility for his or her own pump, continuous glucose monitor (CGM), and diabetes management requires both of you to work together on this important goal. In some instances, parents may be reluctant to give more responsibility to their children, and some children may be hesitant to take it. Other parents may be anxious to turn over responsibility, sometimes even when the child is not ready to assume it. The goal is to encourage, support, and facilitate your child doing what he or she is able to and what should be done with managing diabetes, the pump, and CGM.

Children of all ages can begin to participate in their own care according to their abilities and developmental capabilities. Doing this will lead to the ultimate goal of enabling the young adult to leave home—when the time comes—and be able to manage his or her diabetes safely and effectively. By offering your encouragement and help all along the way, expecting your child to do what is appropriate for his or her age, and supporting your child in doing it, you will prepare him or her for eventual autonomy.

SPECIAL ISSUES FOR ADOLESCENTS AND YOUNG ADULTS

It can be particularly hard for adolescents and young adults to adjust to the rigors of the diabetes regimen. This is because they don't want to be different. They want to lead a "normal" life, and they want to start taking care of themselves more and more. Although diabetes cannot stand in the way of increasing independence and autonomy, diabetes cannot be ignored either. Having an insulin pump and a CGM may make it easier or harder, depending on what the issues are for the individual and his or her family. There are many things to consider, ranging from physiological (physical functions) to psychological (mental functions). Teens and young adults need encouragement, supervision, and even involvement in their lives and diabetes care.

Physiological Issues

The changes in hormone levels and rapid physical growth that occur during puberty increase insulin resistance. When coupled with an increase in calorie intake, which is normal to meet the physical demands of growth, children in puberty may need to significantly increase their insulin dosages, adjust for the dawn phenomenon, and increase the number of times they bolus each day. Menstruation may result in changes in insulin dosages, too. Some girls see high glucose levels before they get their period every month, and they often aren't aware of the reason.

Psychological Issues

The psychological issues that arise during adolescence are often centered on issues of independence. Driving, staying out late, sleeping over at friends' houses, and going off to summer programs and camps, and eventually college, make it imperative that the adoles-

Diabetes Skills and Knowledge by Developmental Age

Age	Skills	Knowledge
Birth to 3 years	• Rapid changes in cognitive and motor skills, nutrition requirements, sleep/wake patterns, and acquisition of developmental milestones	• Inherent trust in parents/caregivers
3–5 years	• Lack motor skills and cognitive ability	• Minimal understanding of diabetes procedures and management issues • Start to ask about food
6–9 years	• Help insert pump catheter • Wear pump appropriately • Protect the catheter site • Unhook pump to give to supervising adult • Reconnect pump, with assistance • Activate bolus dose, with direction	• Understand glucose numbers • Understand importance of blood glucose control • Minimally explain diabetes • Ask about food • May feel different from peers
10–12 years	• Protect pump during activity • Be responsible for pump when unhooked • Insert pump catheter • Hook and unhook pump • Activate bolus dose	• Count carbs • Start to calculate insulin dose for meals and corrections using bolus calculator • Understand that exercise leads to lows
13–14 years	• Suspend basal dose • Program basal rates, with assistance	• Calculate and deliver bolus • Understand the role of exercise • Recognize if basal rates need to be adjusted
15–18 years	• Program changes in basal rates	• Determine what factors affect basal rates and how to check • Determine what new basal rates should be given, with assistance • Determine what factors affect bolus doses • Change algorithm for bolus doses, with assistance • Use sick-day protocol, with assistance

cent and family are in agreement on how they will meet these new challenges. It is also critical that diabetes doesn't become an excuse to hold the teen back from the normal processes of increasing independence. It is equally important that the teen realize that he or she has to effectively manage diabetes to gain and deserve more independence and autonomy.

Driving

Being able to drive is a great milestone and achievement. But driving is also dangerous and can be more dangerous if glucose levels aren't managed. Driving is a privilege that must be earned by gaining experience behind the wheel, learning the rules, and passing a test. For someone with diabetes, it must be earned by showing that glucose control and monitoring are done consistently and reliably before getting behind the wheel. Testing glucose or checking CGM values and rate of change of glucose before driving can help keep everyone safe. Don't forget to have glucose tabs or juice in the car at all times.

Alcohol

Drinking alcohol is different for people with diabetes. Alcohol can have a profound effect on glucose levels and must only be consumed by adults (it is illegal for underage teens to drink). However, even though it is illegal, many teens (even younger ones) drink alcohol, and some do it more than just rarely.

Alcohol can lead to both hyperglycemia and hypoglycemia. Certain alcoholic drinks contain a lot of carbohydrate because they are mixed with fruit juices or sugary sodas or because they contain carbohydrate themselves (beer and sweet wines). Mixers can elevate glucose levels soon after drinking. It is best to avoid covering for these carbohydrates because alcohol has a tendency to cause hypoglycemia later. Alcohol reduces glucose release from the liver and can lead to hypoglycemia between meals and overnight. To compensate, you should eat a snack or meal when you drink and not take insulin for the carbohydrates or at least reduce your insulin dose significantly. Increased monitoring, changing low glucose alerts so you will be informed earlier, waking up in the middle of the night to check your glucose (either by self-monitoring your glucose or by looking at your sensor) and checking your overall health status, and telling friends about the effects of alcohol can help make it safe to drink in moderation (drinking in excess is defined as having more than 1 drink a day for women and more than 2 drinks a day for men).

CHAPTER REVIEW

➡ The tasks required for insulin pump therapy and continuous glucose monitoring increase as a child ages and gains experience with diabetes. Some parents find it hard to give up any responsibility for diabetes care, whereas others can't wait to give their child more responsibility, sometimes when the child is not ready or able. Parents should issue new responsibilities based on your child's development and abilities. By offering your encouragement and help, as well as considering what diabetes tasks your child is prepared for and ready to take on, you can help ensure a safe transition to adulthood.

➡ Teens need supervision, encouragement, and parental involvement in their lives, as well as in their diabetes management.

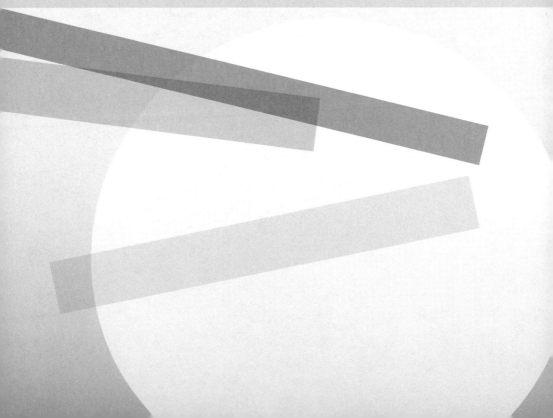

IN THIS CHAPTER

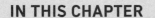

CHAPTER 17

ATTITUDES ABOUT
THE PUMP AND CGM

Adapting to life with the insulin pump and a continuous glucose monitor (CGM) can be difficult and have an effect on your day-to-day mood and ability to succeed with diabetes management. Learning all that you can about the mechanics of the pump and measuring interstitial glucose is different from psychologically dealing with the pump and CGM. Adjusting to diabetes technology can be difficult and take time. With systems that automate insulin delivery, learning to trust the devices that are stopping, and now also giving, insulin is a process for the patient. For many, when the positives and negatives of diabetes technology are carefully weighed, the positives come out on top.

One major issue for every user of diabetes technology is to decide who should know about the devices and when and how to show or tell them. The scenarios for family, friends, and strangers are different. Here are some things to think about when considering the reluctance or hesitancy you may feel about sharing that you wear a pump and a sensor.

OVERALL ATTITUDES

Having diabetes, adjusting to a chronic illness with a complex treatment regimen, and experiencing hypoglycemia and hyperglycemia can be difficult. People go through several emotions—denial, anger, and depression—especially when first diagnosed. For some people, these emotions come back over and over again. Starting on an insulin pump or CGM can bring back these emotions. There is a physi-

DETECT DEPRESSION

If your feelings are affecting your day-to-day living, then you need to discuss this with your diabetes team. People with diabetes have higher rates of depression. Get help. It can make a world of difference!

cal thing attached to the body that serves as a constant reminder that you have diabetes. If you have these emotions, it is important to talk to your diabetes team. Discuss your feelings with them and see if you need to talk to a psychologist, psychiatrist, or social worker. Talk to your parents, other family members, and friends, too. Talking to people close to you can help, even though they might not know what it feels like to have diabetes. They can still listen and offer support.

In addition, try to find a way to talk to others who are like you, with diabetes and a pump and a sensor. Find a support group, go to a diabetes event, read blogs, join Facebook groups, watch YouTube videos (or post some yourself), search for others at your college or join one of the college networks, or go to a diabetes camp (as a camper or counselor). Taking these step will help you feel like you are not alone.

Approach pump therapy with an open mind. Be sure it is right for you. Do the same with a CGM. Work with your family and your health care team. Establish good habits. Make this new part of your journey the best, and then step back and see how much you have learned and hopefully how much better your diabetes management has become.

HOW TO TELL OTHERS ABOUT YOUR PUMP AND CGM

Friends and Family

One of the first things you'll have to decide is how the people who are close to you, such as friends and family, will play a role in your pump and CGM therapy. If you live with a friend, spouse, parent, or significant other, encourage him or her to come to pump and CGM training sessions and learn about diabetes technology. Tell them about automated features if you are using them. This will be helpful if you become ill or have an emergency.

You also need to decide how you want the people with whom you live and interact to assist you with your diabetes. Do you want them to help you remember to bolus before meals, to test often, or to change your infusion set? Or would you prefer that they just know what to do in an emergency? Diabetes is a hard disease to live with if you don't have support, so don't be afraid to ask for help. Everyone needs it!

Your friends and family may be nervous about your diabetes technology at the beginning. Giving them a quick demonstration or information about the pump, CGM, and automated features might make them feel more confident. You need to discuss what you want help with and how to handle an emergency.

Acquaintances and Strangers

If you prefer to conceal your pump and CGM from acquaintances and strangers, then you should be able to do that. However, if the devices are in sight, people may ask what they are. Have a response ready. People may mistake the pump or the receiver for something else, like a cell phone. At functions where cell phones or cameras are prohibited, you may be asked to turn it off or leave it outside. A brief explanation is usually all that is needed. You can say something like, "This it is not a cell phone/camera, but actually an insulin pump or sugar information receiver for my diabetes. These are lifesaving medical devices that I need to keep on me at all times to avoid becoming very ill." If your cell phone is your CGM receiver, there may be issues attending events that ban cameras and phones. Be sure you understand what you need to bring so that you can have

NEED HELP? GOT QUESTIONS?

Call your doctor, nurse, diabetes educator, or the pump or CGM company. They all want to help you succeed with your devices!

CGM Advantages and Disadvantages

Advantages	Disadvantages
Alerts and alarms	Attached to a device
Alerts and alarms warning of glucose values at or predicted to be at a low or high threshold	Placement on your body might be difficult
	Have to deal with adhesive tape
	Can lead to excessive alarms—alarm fatigue
Rate of change alarm to alert when rapid changes in glucose levels are occurring, and when there is a rapid increase indicating a missed meal bolus	Might be visible to the public
	Remembering to calibrate
	Can display inaccurate glucose data
Ability with some devices to allow for automation of insulin delivery	Data overload
	Expense of CGM
Less fingerstick glucose measurements	
Fewer SMBG measurements required with CGM, while getting a new glucose level every 5 minutes	
Extensive data	
Extensive data, which might be integrated with insulin pump therapy, is generated by uploading into a computer program that can be used for better insulin dose adjustments	
Lifestyle flexibility	
Like with pumps, you have an advanced tool for glucose monitoring on your body	
Improved diabetes outcomes	

your phone at these events (i.e., a doctor's note stating you have diabetes and your phone is a component of your care).

WEIGHING IT ALL IN THE BALANCE

Balance is the key when dealing with the ups and downs of diabetes technology. Often, the short-term or immediate issues that develop with the pump or CGM can overshadow the potential positive and often long-term advantages gained. It can be hard to be upbeat and positive about the pump and sensor when you're getting used to a new way of life. But don't forget the advantages: alerts, ability to see your trends and patterns, the bolus calculator, automated features, and hopefully very few or no shots!

Negatives
The biggest issues include having something attached to your body, trouble concealing the devices, having to troubleshoot if problems develop, too many alerts and alarms, and forgetting to bolus. Some people are concerned about concealing the pump and sensor as well as the constant hassle of finding a place to put it, especially if they prefer not to reveal that they have diabetes and/or a diabetes device. When the pump and CGM become more of a hassle than an aid, it's nice to know that they're not permanent and that you can take them off and that you have alternatives.

Another thing that people tend to have issues with is remembering to bolus. Sometimes people forget about the bolus or they take their bolus late. Teens and adolescents transitioning to managing their own therapy often have a hard time remembering to bolus on time. Excuses (for anyone, not just teens) often include being too busy, not knowing the carb count, not wanting to bolus in front of friends or peers, or simply forgetting.

It is hard getting into the habit of taking a bolus every time you eat, but it's very important. We also know that taking insulin 15–30 minutes before eating is very effective for reducing after-meal highs and that the insulin pump makes bolusing easy to do. But it is hard to remember all the time. You may have to ease into bolusing before eating by starting with one meal (breakfast is usually the easiest; wake up, test, calibrate the CGM, and bolus for your food and glucose right away, and then get ready and eat breakfast last). It's important that you develop these good habits and stick to them for the best control.

Sometimes people on the pump get too confident or lax about their habits, which may have been very good at one point. They stop counting carbs and just estimate, or they continually forget to bolus or bolus late, or they just stop using the bolus calculator. These habits add up and, over time, can really affect your A1C and overall health. The loss of good habits might also lead people to dislike their pump.

Positives

There are obviously positive aspects about insulin pumps and CGMs, or people wouldn't choose to use them and doctors wouldn't recommend them. These aspects include (and are not limited to) fewer shots and fingersticks, information about glucose excursions before you develop symptoms, and automation of insulin delivery. CGMs and insulin pumps can be used safely and may help prevent hypoglycemia and hyperglycemia.

CHAPTER REVIEW

➡ Adjusting to diabetes and diabetes technology can be challenging. Denial, anger, and depression can recur when you begin an insulin pump and CGM, reminiscent of how you might have felt when you were first diagnosed with diabetes. Involve others and, if need be, get help from a mental health professional.

➡ Talk to others and involve them in understanding your issues with diabetes and with your insulin pump and CGM.

➡ When you think of the negatives, remember all of the positives about your diabetes devices. Negatives can include always being attached to a machine as a constant reminder of diabetes, the devices making your diabetes more visible, higher risk of ketones if something malfunctions, and the expense of pumps and CGMs. Positives include the reduced number of shots and fingersticks you must take, the decreased likelihood of hypoglycemia and hyperglycemia, and the increased flexibility in your schedule.

CHAPTER 18

LOOKING TO THE FUTURE

Over the last 35 years, there have been remarkable advances in insulin pump therapy. Over the last 15 years, the same can be said for continuous glucose monitoring. These advances have enabled approximately 750,000 people around the world to benefit from using insulin pumps and hundreds of thousands of people have benefitted from continuous glucose monitoring. Systems that automate insulin delivery—threshold-suspend, predictive low glucose management, and hybrid closed-loop systems—have all been approved for commercialization. Data have been generated that show these systems are safe and capable of improving glucose control. But the ultimate promise of diabetes technology has yet to be realized— the fully automated delivery of insulin through an artificial pancreas.

COMPONENTS OF THE ARTIFICIAL PANCREAS

The components of an artificial pancreas would include devices similar to what we have today in hybrid closed-loop systems that require the patient to do meal boluses. The pumps and sensors used now are likely adequate for an artificial pancreas, but modifications and advancements would be required to give all basal and bolus insulin through the artificial pancreas system.

To automatically dose for meals and hyperglycemia (actual or predicted), artificial pancreas systems would have to detect that a person had started to eat or drink calories as soon as glucose starts to elevate. The algorithm would ramp up insulin delivery; however, with present-day rapid-acting insulin preparations, there is an unacceptable delay in insulin absorption and action. Therefore, the development of more rapid or ultra rapid-acting insulin preparations might be a prerequisite for fully closed-loop systems.

Despite major breakthroughs, there are still many questions to answer concerning the artificial pancreas.

What Is the Best Algorithm?

Closed-loop algorithms are being used now in a number of other closed-loop systems, such as the automatic pilot in planes, the thermostat in your house, and the cruise control in your car. A lot of research is being done to develop effective, safe algorithms that can be used in the artificial pancreas.

Is Delivering Only Insulin Sufficient?

Does the artificial pancreas truly have to mimic how the pancreas functions and also have the ability to give glucagon to prevent hypoglycemia? Would the system benefit from giving another hormone, such as pramlintide or a glucagon-like peptide-1 (GLP-1) analog, since both decrease after-meal glucose rises? Pramlintide (from the beta-cell) and GLP-1 (from the intestinal tract) are hormones that are currently used to treat diabetes, and it is possible that they may improve glucose management for people using the artificial pancreas. Conceptually, any of these other hormones might only need to be given intermittently (such as glucagon when the glucose level is falling or pramlintide when a meal is being ingested). Therefore, a pump used in the artificial pancreas may require two chambers (one for insulin and one for the other hormone), or two separate pumps may be needed.

Is the Insulin Now Used Good Enough?

You know that your rapid-acting insulin still acts much more slowly than the insulin released from the pancreas. This result occurs because there is still a delay in its absorption from your subcutaneous tissue, and its main site of action—your liver—is far away. Several strategies could accelerate insulin action to create an effective artificial pancreas. These include newer, more rapid-acting insulins; new developments in infusion sets; and delivering insulin into the abdominal cavity to get closer to the liver.

CONCLUSION

Over the last few decades, we have witnessed incredible advances in diabetes therapies: new rapid-acting insulins; smaller, faster glucose meters; information management with uploaded data from glucose monitors, pumps, and sensors; next-generation pumps and sensors; and devices capable of automating insulin delivery, including threshold-suspend, predictive low glucose management, and hybrid closed-loop systems . We have come a long way, and the reality of a full artificial pancreas is essentially within sight. The end result will be the near-perfect control of glucose levels without much human intervention. We owe thanks to the diabetes associations, including the American Diabetes Association (ADA), the Helmsley Trust, Close Concerns, and the Juvenile Diabetes Research Foundation (JDRF); to the National Institutes of Health; and to many investigators and researchers around the world. But most importantly, we owe thanks to each of you. Those of you who strive to manage diabetes, who use advanced therapies and technologies to get the best results, and who wait for each step on the road to the artificial pancreas.

CHAPTER REVIEW

➡ The artificial pancreas—the fully closed-loop system—will not require as much patient interaction as the hybrid closed-loop system that is available now. By advancing the algorithm, using a more rapidly absorbed insulin, and perhaps by adding another hormone, the artificial pancreas should be able to automatically dose basal and most, if not all, bolus insulin.

➡ In conclusion, much is owed to you; your health care providers; the insulin, pump, and CGM companies; and to researchers across the globe, in addition to diabetes associations, such as the ADA, for enabling us to get to the advances described in this book.

INDEX

Note: Page numbers in **bold** indicate an in-depth discussion on the topic